Get in Trouble!

Stories from classrooms of the
Freedom Writer Teachers

Torbjørn Ydegaard (Ed.)

Get in Trouble!

Stories from classrooms of the
Freedom Writer Teachers

Colophon

©Torbjørn Ydegaard and the contributors, 2016
Get in Trouble! Stories from classrooms of the Freedom Writer Teachers

Publisher: BoD – Books on Demand, Copenhagen, Denmark
Production: BoD – Books on Demand GmbH - Norderstedt, Germany

ISBN: 9788771705706

Content

Quincy Murdock
- We get into trouble　　　　　7

Meridith Akuhata-Brown
- Trouble　　　　　8

Alphonso Amos
- Always in Trouble　　　　　11

Tara Bordeaux
- The Ride　　　　　16

CarolAnn Edscorn
- Lacking　　　　　27

Bill Feaver
- Beauty in Inevitable!　　　　　36

Barb Fouts-Melnychuk
- Leaving a Legacy Behind: So many months wasted!　　　　　46

Lisa Liss
- LineGame Problems　　　　　57

Richard Mellot
- For my students　　　　　65

Anne Schober
- Close Your Door – Open Your Heart　　　　　71

Marcus Strother
- Getting in trouble for me　　　　　77

Henry Wright
- A better life through education　　　　　86

Torbjørn Ydegaard, with Kathrin Schaller, Dennis Röben and Frederik Wärn Pedersen
- Freedom Writers in the Arctic　　　　　93

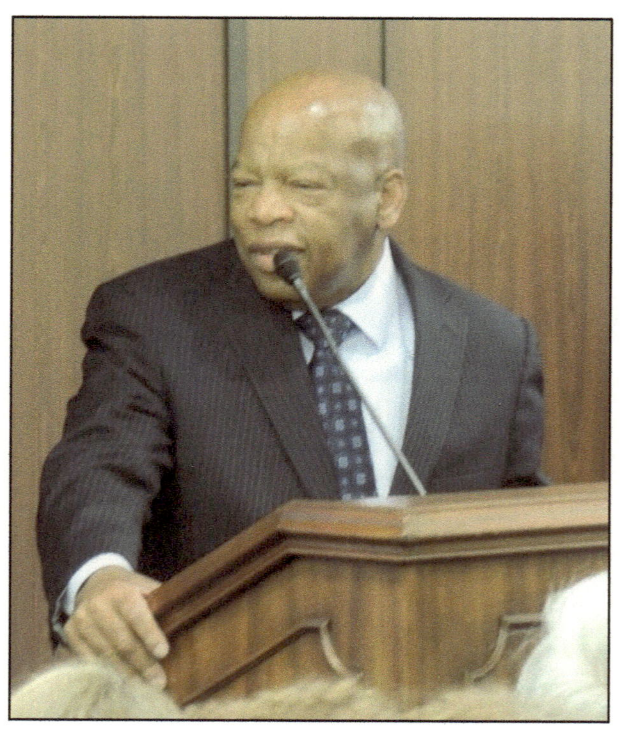

In honor of Rep. John Lewis, who taught us to "get in trouble!"
And so we do!

WE get into trouble,
break down the walls of oppression, kicking aside the rubble.
Teaching what needs to be taught,
many hard battles, have, and will be fought.
The start to getting into positive trouble is to change your negative thoughts.
So much passion in our movement, we are the iron that fire wrought.
The struggle for equality, and meaningful education cannot be bought.

Unjust judgments
some police are brutal,
fighting social inequalities alone is futile.
But just like fingers, when made into a fist,
there is power in unity, light and righteousness must exist
Seeing our youth excel and reach their goals and dreams is our wish.

Many want to see through glasses the color of rose,
but a few of us have been chose
to fight the good fight, courageously run this race,
keep pace.

Despite the setbacks

Spirit has no lack,
ignorance and prejudice we beat back.

A man: his last name Lewis, his first name was John,
Said getting in trouble was the true way to make progress,
being passive is a con
Love for humanity is indeed the magic wand.

– Quincy Murdock

Meridith Akuhata-Brown

Trouble

After I trained as a Freedom Writer Teacher I have been able to share my experiences in local classrooms where I have used some of the Freedom Writer methods.

One classroom I had the opportunity to share my freedom writer experiences was at a local boy's high school in a classroom of year 12 students. Year 12 or 6th Form in New Zealand generally means students are 16-17 years of age.

This particular classroom I had previously taught some health education too so I was known to the students and we had a positive rapport.

I decided that because we had a good rapport and knew a little about each other that I would lead the "line game" with the students and unpack some of the emotions and impacts this activity has on individuals and the whole classroom.

When I arrived into the classroom I noticed that the students were all sitting in their ethnic groups, which for Gisborne means mainly Maori and Pakeha (of European or British decent). There were a couple of students from Vanuatu in this classroom also.

So I started the day asking the boys if they were comfortable enough to go and sit next to someone they had never sat next to before. The boys were happy to oblige me and they all moved to sit next to someone of another ethnicity. I asked them how they felt and they all generally agreed they felt fine. So I began a general discussion around the choices they make and what makes them hold these views. Most of the students didn't realize that they chose each day to sit with the same ethnic group and really did this unconsciously. Some students did notice the pattern and assumed it was the way the class functioned so followed suit.

The discussion lead to unpacking some of the decisions we make either consciously or unconsciously and why we make them, many of the students were genuinely interested in what made them choose and they unpacked some values held by themselves and their families.

We then went into the "line game" and I started with some basic social questions such as step to the line if you are the eldest child, middle child and youngest child, step to the line if you live with two parents, single parent either mum, dad, other etc. Step to the line if you had breakfast this morning.

Some of the questions were in line with some of the issues we are facing here in NZ around the number of single parented families and also the rise in the number of students that come to school hungry.

As we worked through the questions the students became quieter and a sense of solidarity was noticeable. I ventured further into some deeper social issues and asked "step to the line if you have a family member in Jail/Prison" a couple of students stepped forward, at this a couple of students' facial expressions and quiet gasps showed they were shocked but it seemed to send the message "you don't know what others are going through" and a sense of empathy filled the room.

My final questions were "step to the line if you have ever thought about suicide" sadly the majority of the class stepped forward. I then asked them to "step forward if you have ever spoken to someone when you were feeling down/low". Only two boys stepped forward, both pakeha.

This unfortunately reaffirmed a huge issue we have here in NZ, where we have alarming suicide rates amongst young Maori men and one of the key problems for them is talking to someone about their feelings especially when they are feeling down. Culturally for many young Maori men sharing emotions is not something they do well as it implies they are weak also many of them don't have a father figure to help support them through adolescence.

The teacher in the classroom was actually quite stunned at the honesty and openness of the students and told me he was a little embarrassed about how little he knew about them and their lives. We discussed the need to investigate the school's role in supporting the students and a need to share some of the learning's of the day with the guidance department.

Alphonso Amos
Always in Trouble

Anytime you attempt to place academics over athletics, you will automatically get yourself in trouble. In my community sports means everything. We have one huge game that is classified as the biggest football game of the year, the Crosstown Showdown, where the two rival high schools in my city face off against each other. Every year as the game approaches, I cannot stop thinking about the hype of the game. I enjoy watching our students from both Port Huron High and Port Huron Northern High School battle it out on the field, however knowing many of the struggles of our athletes and their ability to get into college is heartbreaking. The numbers of area students who play sports and then go off to college after high school graduation and succeed are not as elevated as some might expect.

We continue to attempt to resolve the issues regarding why only 13% of our community have obtained Bachelor's Degrees and why our students are not prepared to attend community college. I suggest that we wander down a path that is traditionally left unexamined because of its sensitive nature. In fact, as I write these words, I am already contemplating the need to change my name, phone number and e-mail address; delete my Facebook and town because of the overwhelming number of emails and phone calls I will receive telling me that I just do not understand how important this route really is to our children's development.

I am talking about sports and the amount of time and energy our students are dedicating to it while we are failing them academically. Just like my community, there are many others who struggle with similar issues. It often seems like it is a battle between athletics and academics when in reality they both should go hand and hand.

In many communities, we place blame on the teachers, parents and students when instead the problem with academically struggling athletes are the individuals in the community that don't offer support. We are generally the problem. That is right, I said what many would not agree with; we are failing our students. Many of you may be wondering, "What exactly does he mean by WE? My child does not attend school here. That is a school district issue not mine. I do not work in the schools, how am I failing the students?"

When addressing the issue of failed academics among our athletes or any student in that case we are all to blame. It often blows my mind to see the amount of people who come out rivalry games and other athletic events because I know how hard it is to get parents to come to informational meetings, and business and community leaders to mentor or tutor a child. Yet when it's time for the Big Game, everyone jumps on board and supports our students. Large numbers of alumni attend the events in droves, and yet, they ignore the fact that the success of today's students is even more vital than in the past. They are our future. It is their legacy we must be concerned with.

We have allowed sports to oversee academics in so many ways. Working in the area of youth development and education, I have seen firsthand the lack of time our students who play sports have left over to really focus on their academics. Many times students will miss opportunities for tutoring, college advising, SAT Prep and many other academic services because they are going straight to practice after school. Our football players miss out on summer academic camps such as STEM, Career Navigation, Leadership and so many more life changing opportunities.

While writing this article one story comes to mind. I call it the story of lost hope. A previous student in a program I worked in while an employee at SONS Outreach left a void in my heart because of the pressure they received from coaches to be at the "mandatory" practices. In my opinion, no athlete should have to choose sports over something that will help advance him or her academically. This particular student (who will remain nameless) played multiple sports for four years while at Port Huron High School. Many teachers allowed this athlete to sleep in class and barely coast by. Coaches encouraged him, applauding his athletic ability while academically he was failing. He would often times make the newspaper and the community would rally around his ability to do well on the playing field. His hopes and dreams of going attending college after high school was quickly sidelined.

During his senior year that hope began to fade. He had failed to do well in class. Because of his concentration in sports, he had little time to prepare to study for the ACT test so his score was low, yet coaches continued to whisper in his ear that he had the potential to be recruited by a college to play football or basketball. As senior year began to come to an end I discovered that over thirty schools were interested in picking this student up to play for them, however, by the time the staff in our program started working with him it was too late. Many of the schools who were interested could not even consider accepting him because of his low academic achievement. I was livid. How could the educators responsible for shaping his future allow this young man to slip through the cracks? This situation caused me to wonder how many more students we are failing.

As I began to research and engage with parents of athletes, I was in awestruck at the number of parents who have no idea what colleges are looking for in student athletes. In addition to that, many of the students in our area appear to not even be prepared to attend a community college. Yet every year we continue to rally around sports organizing huge tailgating events to raise money, all while our students fall by the wayside.

We teach our students to value what is important by the importance we attach to it. We often fail to stress the same importance for academics as we do for sports. Imagine if we held a huge citywide pep rally, held a tailgate party with bands playing and crowds cheering, celebrating the academic achievements of all of the students. Our enthusiasm and support would honor all those who excel academically and completely change the mindset of the students to shift from athlete to student athlete while we honor those students whose interests may not include sports but whose interest in academics would be recognized as equally important.

Imagine the numbers on jersey being the GPA and ACT/SAT score of the students. I wonder how embarrassed we all would feel when the harsh reality of how we are failing our students is openly displayed for the public to see. Would we cheer for those who represent the number 1.5 or would we applaud only those displaying the numbers 2.5 and above. When high school is over, what do these young athletes have? Memories of winning a game will not get our students admitted to college.

I am not one that just states the problems. I believe in solutions. We as a community are a part of that solution. Restaurant owners, you can encourage students to achieve academically by offering promotions like a discount on a meal for good report cards. Community leaders, you can tutor or mentor a student. Academic leaders, we must find time after school for those athletes to be able to get the educational services they need to excel.

Most importantly parents, you have to make yourself aware of what your child needs to succeed in the future. It is vital that you take time to visit with college and career advisers, meet with the high school counselors and get a solid understanding on what your student is struggling with. In order for us to create great student athletes, we have to remember that they are students first. When academics are the first priority, we build a great student athlete. I believe that by working together we can support our students by helping them achieve in every aspect in their life. That will require everyone to do their part.

Tara Bordeaux
The Ride

They say you never forget your first, but I think that statement is slightly erroneous. It's too vague. Your first *what?* First love? Probably. Heartbreak? That's even more probable. First toy maybe? It's highly unlikely, but not impossible. I could go on and on with this line of questioning, but the truth is that generic sentence should, in the very least, say you never forget your *firsts*, not first. Disagree? Then try it for yourself. Ask yourself about all the firsts in your life, and see where it takes you. I bet you start recalling a plethora of moments you embarked on a different path, met someone new, tried a new food, or just plain started something for the first time. The significance of those events, and whether or not those experiences have a positive or negative impact, is all about perception.

For most of us, there is so much excitement, mystery, and eagerness in initiating something for the first time, we get completely caught up in the moment, inadvertently neglecting the unspoken convention that every new beginning comes from some other beginning's end. For some, that really isn't a big deal, but for others, if not careful, the weight of change between an ending and a beginning becomes a Pandora's box that once opened cannot be resealed. That seems to be the proverbial story of my life. A non-stop revolving door of starts and stops in my own personal inferno that even Dante himself refuses to walk through.

It's like that awful carnival ride, the Tilt-a-Whirl, my mother made me ride with her as a child. It just spun around and around and around, and every time I thought it was the end of the ride,

I'll be damned if it didn't start over again. It was nauseating, and I hated it. But every year, I rode it with her, no scratch that, *for* her, because I loved her so much the thought of letting her down was too much for my little heart to comprehend. Now here I am, thirty years later, wondering why I ever put myself through all of that. Why did I do something that made me anxious, sick, and ready to run away from my life? The only logical answer I come up with is love. I did it for *love*.

When I see it written like that on paper, it seems inspiring, almost admirable, and sacrificial, but I know deep down that is far from the truth. I've made too many mistakes to be "admirable," and I know I have given my mother enough hell in her life that to be fair, she may have put me on that ride so I could feel what it was like for her to deal with me. I was trouble. I could never make good decisions, and when I screwed up and took a wrong turn, which I inevitably did frequently, instead of putting the brakes on the car, I hit the gas and drove as far away from my mistakes as I could. So far, in fact, that I drove all the way to Los Angeles from Dallas just to escape my life, which was the first of many non-stop trips between California and Texas in what has now become my present day carnival ride that never stops spinning.

When I moved to Los Angeles in 2004 to pursue a career in filmmaking as a writer, I thought I had finally found what I was missing in my life. I fell completely and utterly in love with California in a way I have never loved anything else in my life. Cali was my *first* true love. It became a part of me. The more I learned to navigate through Hollywood, the more successful I became in the film industry, and the closer I came to being a writer, I felt like for the first time ever, I was home. I told my friends, my family, and myself I would never leave Cali, never leave Los Angeles, and never leave the film industry.

But you know how the word "never" works, right? The minute you say you are *never* going to do something, or something is *never* going to happen, the universe smacks you in the back of the head and before you know it, you are steering the Titanic through the icebergs wishing you *never* said it was unsinkable. My maiden voyage moment happened when my life in Cali came to a screeching halt. After six weeks in the hospital, five major surgeries, and near death, I needed a break from the 7 days a week, 12-15 hour workdays that were slowly killing me. That conclusion however, took two years for me to finally make the heartbreaking decision to leave LA, and take a position teaching filmmaking in Austin.

As I packed up my studio, I told myself I was never going to leave Cali permanently, it would just be for a year, and I would come back home. I loaded up the last of the boxes in my car, and took one more look around the loft, carefully memorizing every detail of the place I called home for both work and pleasure for the last 8 years, then slowly made my way to the window. I stared out into the most beautiful nighttime skyline view of downtown Los Angeles, and listened to the sounds of the city, fully believing it was telling me not to go. Trying to hold back the tears that began streaming down my face, I was overwhelmed with pain. For the first time in my life, I didn't want to run, but I had to, and before I knew it, I was back on the road again, heading back to the state I so fanatically left almost ten years earlier.

When the first day of teaching arrived, I was nervous, yet strangely confident. I was teaching in a Title I school in one of the roughest parts of Austin, and the naïve filmmaker in me, whose only experience in teaching came from watching movies like *Dangerous Minds* and *Freedom Writers*, thought inspiring students would be as easy as a few fist pumps and a bag of candy. I have no idea what made me think that, seeing that I was a high school dropout who knew students like myself needed much more than that. Nevertheless, I went into that first day thinking I had it in the bag, but within a few hours, I was ready to pack up and run back to Cali as fast as I could. My first day of teaching gave me hot flashes, vomiting, and things I'm not even comfortable typing about. In summary, it was awful.

The very first student to ever talk to me, Johnathan, scared the crap out of me. He walked directly to where I was standing, got pretty close to my face, and with the most intense look in his eyes, and a deepness in his voice that sounded more like a grown man than a freshman in high school said, "what are we doing today Miss?" That simple sentence took every ounce of my confidence and threw it out of the building. I froze, because the truth was, I had no idea what I was doing, and in an instant, felt like a fraud, and he was not the kind of student you wanted to appear to be a fake too. I handed him my carefully planned 22 pages syllabus, (yes, 22 pages, stop laughing), and told him "we are going to cover this." He looked at the packet, looked back at me, and shook his head as he found a seat in the back of the room.

The next two months of my first year of teaching were a blur. I barely connected to my students, and spent more time redirecting them, or telling them to get off their phones, and stop talking then actually teaching them about filmmaking. Some students, like Johnathan, just did not speak at all. They had no respect for me, or themselves, and I hated teaching. I didn't want to be there. I was so frustrated trying to plan lessons, take certification classes to become a highly qualified teacher, and mess with all of the ridiculous red tape that goes into teaching at a public school, just to have students not care or be interested in class. I was over it. I called my best friend and told her, "That's it. I'm done." She laughed a little before making fun of me for wanting to quit so easily. She spent a good half hour unsuccessfully trying to remind me why I wanted to teach for a year in the first place, before finally giving up and saying, "maybe you should quit." Needless to say, she hit my stubborn side and I went back the next day.

A short time after that conversation, one of the original Freedom Writers, Manny Scott, spoke at our school, and his words were all the students could talk about for a while. A good majority of my low performing students were now riding the positive train and trying really hard to do better, but as fast as they got on track, they were abruptly derailed when one of their peers took his own life on campus during lunch. It was the first time for most of them to experience suicide and death, and for some of the most unfortunate students, it was the first time to see a dead body. The death of a student shook both students and teachers to the core, and changed the course of the entire year.

When students returned to school the next day, every class, every student, sat in complete silence. They didn't want to talk, they weren't on their phones, and it was eerily quiet. I looked around the room at the first class that I had since the incident, and realized that I was lost for words, too. As they pulled out their composition books to get ready for the day, I had an overwhelming voice in my head that kept reminding me of the *Freedom Writers* film, and how writing in journals changed the lives of the students in Ms. G.'s class. I knew that after hearing Manny, and seeing the film, the stories of the Freedom Writers were still fresh in their minds, and that maybe it was time to change the composition books from note taking devices to journals.

I started talking about the Freedom Writers, and how they used journals to deal with the painful things they were dealing with in their lives, and asked my students to raise their hands if they would like to use their composition books for journaling that day instead. Tears began to fill my eyes when every hand in the room slowly started to inch up, and I knew that what was happening in my classroom was bigger than I was ready for. Class after class, the same thing happened. The students wanted to write. They wanted to have a voice, be heard, and be able to express themselves and what they were feeling. Even Johnathan, who barely spoke to me, raised his hand.

As the students began writing in their journals every day, I learned more and more about them and what they were going through in their lives. I read all kinds of stories, some short and sweet, some funny, and some absolutely heartbreaking. I learned about their favorite things like food, music, movies, clothing, video games, and more. I read about the people they were crushing on, the ones they were dating, or who just broke up with them. I found out that several of my students were homeless or living in motels, some were living without electricity, many of them could not afford water for showers, some were having problems with parents, several were LGBT and struggling, and some were even thinking about ending their own life. It was overwhelming, but I read 150 journals word for word, and commented back on every one of them.

The more they wrote, the more they opened up to me, and me to them. We laughed more in class. They put their phones up when asked. Even Johnathan was different. He no longer sat in the back of the class silent. Instead, he moved his desk next to mine, and spent every morning before school, and every day at lunch in my classroom. He wrote lyrics in his journal, and wanted to learn how to make music for his words, so I gave him the software, an instruction manual and let him go at it. It was a complete turnaround for my students and I, and somewhere in that transitional period, I no longer hated teaching. I loved my students deeply, and I could tell that even though they didn't say it, they loved me back.

When the last day of school came that first year, I gave all of my students little cards with candy bags, and personally told each of them goodbye. We took pictures, laughed, and made more memories. It wasn't until Jonathan, while standing with a group of students signing my yearbook said, "Miss, I can't *wait* to take your class next year," that my heart fell out of my chest. One after another students agreed with him, and the more excited they got about coming to school the following year, I more I wanted to run out of that room. How could I tell these kids that I was just like everyone else? That I could just walk out and leave just like that? How could I not only disappoint them, but the principle that hired me that I respected so dearly? Where was my loyalty? I felt a pain in my heart that I hadn't felt since the day I walked out of my studio in LA. Once again, I was in trouble. I was in another one of my infamous decision making moments and the outlook wasn't looking good.

As I contemplated back and forth about leaving, I kept the keys to my classroom over the summer, and spent most of my time cleaning the room and setting it up for the next teacher. (Yes, *teacher*, not *year*.) It wasn't until August, when I attended the Freedom Writers Institute in Long Beach, that I started to realize the importance of what I was doing. I started thinking about Johnathan, and all of my other students, and I knew I had to go back at least one more year, to finish what I started. It felt euphoric, and I was inspired to take my passion for film and pass it on to my students. I returned to school, flames burning to see my kids again, and to meet the new bunch coming in. And sure enough, just like my first year, Johnathan was the first one at my door that morning ready to go.

It was a crazy year. My kids and I grew closer, and my heart grew for them as fast as the Grinch's on the hill. Johnathan took his love of music to the next level, writing lyrics, creating beats, and even getting up in front of the school and rapping at lunchtime. He put together a lunchtime crew of freestylers, who would come to my room to battle, and he even created an old school hip hop song titled, "Ms.B.," named after one of his favorite teachers. Go figure. He was on top of the world, and so was I. I promised him that by his senior year, we would make sure there was a music studio added to the film program for him and the rap crew to make real tracks in. That's when iceberg number two hit.

Midway through the year, Johnathan walked into my classroom for the last time. He came to tell me goodbye, because he had to leave school after a fall out with his family. It was heartbreaking. We fought back the tears, both of us too hard to admit saying goodbye was too painful, so instead, we just fist pumped and half hugged it out. I handed him a mic from my drawer, and told him to keep making music, and change the world the way he changed me. He shook his head in disbelief, and gave me a partial wave as he walked out the door, never looking back. My heart broke in a way I can't explain. My first student to ever speak to me, spoke to me for the last time. I wanted to help, to save him from what was happening, but I couldn't. I had no idea how to.

After losing my first student, I spent the rest of that year trying to "save" every other student I could, even if that meant breaking the rules. But I wasn't the only one. I knew many teachers who truly cared about their kids that did the same type of things I did, like having snacks in the room, extra jackets and blankets, giving rides home when it was unsafe for kids to walk, you name it. We knew the risks involved, but we took them anyway because we knew our kids were worth getting into trouble for.

When I found out one of my students and her siblings, whose mother was very ill, was going to be evicted out of their motel room, I made some calls to buy them time. I didn't care if it was right or wrong to do, my only concern was that she and her family were safe. I brought clothes to school for students and let them take what they wanted. I bought books for them to read outside of class. If they liked one of my toys on my desks, I gave it to them. If they needed a backpack, or supplies, I did my best to always keep my room stocked. I did whatever I could for them, all the while thinking about Johnathan, and hoping wherever he was; someone was looking out for him, too.

It's been over a year since I saw Johnathan, but his influence on my classroom, especially me, is still an everyday presence. When one of my students produced a documentary short on our school librarian for SXSWedu, it was Johnathan's song that played in the closing credits. As my student filmmakers and I sat in the theatre watching our film end, I knew the moment his name rolled through the credits, he would be as proud to see it in lights as I was. Those same students who made the documentary, came to me after with the idea to start a music production studio, to help at-risk students find a safe place to express themselves creatively. I told them I wasn't sure if we could get approval, but they were determined.

They called it *The Lost & Sound Room*, where "lost" students could find themselves and their own voice through music. They believed in the idea so much, they pitched it for a competition where they were semifinalists, and won almost half the funds needed for a start-up studio, then raised the rest of the money online. Their efforts made it into the hands of the right people at SXSW, who generously donated a full blown sound booth. It was a surreal moment, watching my kids do something so important for others.

Seeing the excitement in their faces when they knew they were doing something special, reminded me why I became a teacher. I started out teaching to make a difference, and inspire kids to follow their dreams, make good choices, and stay out of trouble, but it didn't exactly go as planned. Instead, they inspired *me*, taught *me,* and momentarily stopped the ride I've been on from spinning long enough to allow Dante to lead me out of my "it will only be a year" purgatory. They taught me more about sacrificing and love in my short time with them then I ever thought possible, and completely changed my life. So much so, that I started cheating on California, and fell in love with something else.

Next year, marks my fourth year teaching, and what should be Jonathan's senior year. He won't be there on day one to greet me at the door like before, but ironically, just as I promised him, there will be a music studio. Most of my kids have graduated now, and only a handful of my first year students remain. When the school year ends and they graduate next year, I will too. It will be the end of the first set of students for me, and like I said before, you never forget your *firsts*.

Johnathan and those first year students, and every set of students after that year will always be a part of me. The ride may still be spinning, but I don't mind it now. I know that no matter how hard it spins me, eventually I'll get off. I'm not running. I'm not lost, and I'm not making the life-altering bad decisions I made before. For the first time in my life, I am learning to truly follow my heart instead of running from my mistakes, and I could not have learned to do that without knowing each and every one of my students.

Because of them, this writer wrote her *first* published piece, and I will forever be grateful to those kids, and *never* forget the way they touched my heart and changed my life. (Hmm, maybe you can say never after all). Of course, I'll still get into trouble every now and then, because there will always be some rule I'm never supposed to break when it comes to helping others, but we know how that will go, I'll still get into trouble, and I'll still do it for love.

It really is true what they say, that *every new beginning comes from some other beginning's end.*

CarolAnn Edscorn
Lacking

Childhood Memories.
Youth memories.
Adult memories.
Sometimes, I do wonder how I made it to be old.
Yet here I am.

Diagnosed with autism 22 years ago, I initially rejoiced, thrilled to understand that my quirks and oddities have a basis in neurodiversity. Time moved along, and I began meeting parents and educators and autistics. I became troubled in spirit.

Memories, piling up, clouding joy, misdirecting truth. I had to change, had to do, had to find a way, a voice, and a method to my madness.

I began to share and teach. I offer workshops and seminars at conferences around the New England region and the United States.

Today is the first part of a two day educator conference in a rural region, where resources and science based knowledge are scant. I spend hours, days, on developing my workshops. I have to process all those memories as I appraise the topics, the insights and the needs of the school district.

All those memories…

–   'Why can't you act like the other kids?'

–   'What are you doing now?'

–   'Can't you sit still?''

-     'Hello? Anybody in there?'
-     'Pay attention. You're always in your own little world.'
-     'How can someone so smart be so stupid?'
-     'You forgot your chores AGAIN?'

I hear these words in the tones and timbres of many people over decades. They led to deep levels of self-doubt, of self-hatred. I believed them, and they dragged me to suicide.

So I know. Oh yes, I know how important words and emotional energy are in all relationships. And I have to change, have to do, have to find a way, my voice, communicate my story so others have a better life.

It's been a tough morning.

Throughout my workshops I pause and ask participants to share their new understandings, how they might apply concepts of functional behavioral analysis, the tenets of positive behavior supports and strength-based programming. How does knowing more about the sensory integration and processing challenges affect your classroom design? What can you adjust in curriculum delivery knowing about the neuroscience of autism? Are there ways to shift your attitudes, behaviors and language to become a safe haven for youth?

I listen, respectful; simply glad that most can articulate their awareness and propose the changes which can happen.

Yet…not today, no, no longer can my voice remain quiet when I hear this young teacher begin: "I just know I can better help these poor, lost—"

I stand up straight and my hand reaches towards her and my voice erupts: "No. Stop. Please. Why is your student 'poor?'

What is 'lost' about your student? You are not alone in these feelings and words, and I can tell you, they are only lost if you assume they are!"

All those memories flood through my thoughts. I hear the words echoing, instructing me: SHUT UP, CarolAnn, what do you KNOW, how can you SAY THAT?

But I cannot listen to memories when I know that the future of a young person whom I will likely never meet yet depends on finding my courage. I cannot succumb when I can give hope. I have to offer hope through these dedicated educators who have beautiful intentions.

"I ask you to forgive me for interrupting, yet I cannot apologize. Every time a person uses sad words, lost words, empathy words, it tells me that there is an intrinsic belief in limitations. Autistics may not express themselves and their feelings, or do so well, but we do pick up on emotions and energy. There are countless autistic lives, where a gloomy prognosis is overturned simply when communication becomes possible. Often these leaps of love are predicated on new technologies.

I have numerous videos and articles reflecting the abundant diversity in language reception and expression. Let's re-visit a slide from my Introduction."

I scroll back through my power point slides.

Words

–   Disorder
–   Disability
–   Lost
–   Non-verbal

–   Non-compliant

–   Retarded

How do these words make YOU feel? What if they are applied to YOU?

–   What do YOU think of when you hear the word disability?
–   What do YOU think of when you hear the word disorder?
–   What do YOU think of when you hear the word AUTISM?

IT IS A DIAGNOSIS. It is not the whole person,
not the entire story.

"All behavior is communication. All behavior serves a purpose. We might not know the purpose, and we cannot PRESUME to know the purpose either."

I look around the classroom. I try to discern what they are feeling, what they are absorbing. I fail, of course. Facial expressions are not a skill which comes easily to me. But when I first began teaching about autism someone taught me to look and see if the faces are looking toward me.

Sweetness, but looking at faces and eyes takes so MUCH courage! Anxiety threatens to defeat me. But I look and they are, indeed, watching me. I know I can continue!

I also observe that the room is electrically charged, too quiet. The young paraprofessional is still standing, with her hands rubbing together, her skin tone pale.

Breathe, I say to myself. I am not a threat, and my students here are not threats either.

30

I smile. I indicate that she is free to sit again! I. Am. Not. A. Threat.

"So often the emphasis in accommodations and modifications is on changing the child. When behaviors are unexpected, when they don't meet normal and natural expectations, we become uncomfortable, and we look for solutions to this prickly situation.

"Observe. The environment is overwhelming. Relationships are intimidating. The mind and body are in conflict. How can we possibly reduce this alarming state of affairs so that learning can happen? How can we redirect all the psychic and emotional NOISE barriers, so that opportunity can progress?"

I cannot stop smiling! Yet they are all frowning! I think: They are thinking! I move to another set of slides.

"Values, inspiration, and belonging: these are difficult concepts to teach, and even to model. So here is your new mantra, your new song, and your new fundamental guide!

–   Change the environment.
–   Change yourself.
–   Allow the child to change.

Let's say this together, yes?"

And together we speak softly: Change the environment. Change myself. Allow the child to change. I smile bigger.

"Hey, it's new. Let's be a bit bolder?"

I point to the slide. Voices respond. But I don't feel the belief, the affirmation and acknowledgement that radiates when learning becomes internal. My brain is moving through years of books, of insights, of researching studies and of life experience.

"What are some behaviors in autism which we see regularly?"

Answers: rocking, swaying, bouncing, hand flapping. Got it!

I call it hand dancing or hand flying. My hands are wings. It's my internal energy escaping, hoping someday to flee gravity. After bullying and parental "corrections" I learned to keep my dancing hands low, below eye level. But this is a behavior which very often gets addressed as BAD and therefore requiring FIXING, even eliminating.

I sit on top of the desk, cross my legs, and begin shaking my foot. I shake it rapidly, exaggerated.

"So. Hand flapping. It's a bit startling, isn't it?" Heads nod. I let go of some rules. I begin humming. I have near perfect music pitch. I close my eyes, sway my head side to side, and hum a happy slice of music. My hands lift off and I enter my happy zone for a short time. It is so hard to share this after decades of having to hide the behaviors which calm me, lift my spirit, and help me integrate the outer environment, the world, with my interior perspectives.

It's a stimulation pattern, mostly an unconscious effort to have control in a situation which feels out of control. It's been shortened to stimming in daily, informal situations.

"I think it accurate that if I were in public, in a classroom, an airport, a restaurant, I would definitely attract some attention! But really, what is WRONG with this? Does anyone play air guitar any more? Does anyone wave a conductor's wand listening to music, or a wizarding wand to drive away fears? Anyone make the sound effects and take the stance of a Jedi wielding a light saber?"

There are smiles and nods.

"Does anyone have a Dad or friend who jingles coins in the pants pocket?"

More smiles, more acceptance. I smile too!

"Well, will you confess to foot stimming? It's below eye level, low to the ground, out of sight. But I assure you, most of you in this room have waved your feet, pretty enthusiastically, too." I point at the slide again: Change the environment. Change yourself. Allow the child to change.

"Let's try standing up, straight and tall! Let's state this declaration with loud joy! Maybe the staff upstairs will hasten down here to find out what's happening!"

There is something very human about wanting to understand, and to belong. Smiling and laughing they all stand, a bit awkwardly, but together in spirit. I am tempted to invite them to hold hands! But we simply time ourselves:

Change the environment.
Change ourselves.
Allow the child to change.

There are only 20 educators in my workshop. There are 200 plus educators in the school district. I have come back to this district three times in the past three years. The administration is proactive about inclusion and universal design. They include paraprofessionals in the trainings.

How many other schools don't have current information or know what Best Practices are now? Research reveals new information almost daily.

I am not done with this cohort. This is our first day together. Language habits are insidious. I hear it daily.

−	Poor kid. Lost in her own little world.

(Make the world a safer place.)

−	Can't you control your child?

(Can't you control your mouth?)

−	THESE children with disabilities are holding the bright students back.

(No. Studies across the nation and internationally demonstrate that Inclusion is good for all students. It does require some training.)

−	This kid is a loser. Just can't focus on anything.

(Error. They are focusing. On what they want and what makes them happy. How many of us can claim that tenacity?)

−	Autism is an epidemic with its basis in bad parenting.

(Ignorance is contagious, not autism.)

−	I don't trust anyone who can't make eye contact.

(Even toddlers can look you in the eye and LIE about eating the cookies.)

−	Making eye contact is crucial to social success.

(Not in 85% of the tribal and less developed countries and regions. Eye contact is considered rude and an invitation to fight.)

−	Having friends in one's peer group is vital to success.

(Over time we make friends across generations and across demographics. Peer dependency encourages cliques and bullying.)

Change the environment.
Change yourself.
Allow the child to change.

On our lunch break I mosey over to the young paraprofessional whom I interrupted. Her face is one huge smile. Perhaps I truly do not need to apologize? She gazes down at the carpeting.

"I've always felt WRONG somehow, always seeing my students as incomplete or broken. At first I was upset when you called me on it. But as the workshop progresses, I understand how the brain works, how sensory integration can derail learning, how it's the simple things about inclusion and acceptance which changes the classroom. I wouldn't want other people to think of ME as broken or lost, even though I can be spacey or distracted. I feel stronger and happier about being a para. This is great. Thank you."

No words. I simply nod and smile. One convert achieved. Six billion more to go.

END

Bill Feaver

Beauty is Inevitable!

I started teaching at the Fresno County Juvenile Hall in 2000. I taught in the lockdown unit at the old juvenile hall. I had two classes of ten students each. I was looking for ideas and strategies to reach these students.

At my first Fresno County Office of Education All-Staff Day, a young woman named Erin Gruwell was the keynote speaker. Her speech was so intriguing; she was talking about my students. The Freedom Writers Diary was being sold in the foyer. I bought a copy, read it, loved it and bought a class set.

The Freedom Writers Diary was read each year I was in the locked down unit. In the spring of 2005, I attended a reading conference. Again Erin Gruwell was the keynote speaker. She was waiting alone while people came in for the final session. I had my copy of the Freedom Writers Diary all dog-eared, marked up and starting to fall apart. I walked up to Erin, introduced myself and asked if she would autograph my book.

Erin fingered through the book looking it over...her eyes teared. We talked about what and where I taught. She asked many questions about me and she wrote… "Dear Bill, when diverse worlds come together...beauty is inevitable! To the beauty that awaits us... Erin Gruwell, your kindred spirit!" I did not know at the time how true those words were and how close we would become. This was the start of my ride on the Freedom Writer Express!

Erin came to speak at juvenile hall (the old facility) and the boot camp in the fall of 2005; we became family. At the end of

2005 I was invited to be one of the teachers in the first Freedom Writers Institute. We met for three long weekends over 2006 as the Freedom Writer Foundation developed their Teacher Institute. It has been ten years of using the Freedom Writers strategies in varying ways.

A colleague of mine, Michelle Trevino, and I at Worsley School developed two units using some of the Freedom Writers strategies. The units were developed to coincide with Banned Book Week. One unit was used in my Language Arts class and the other in my history class. Because the Freedom Writers Diary has been banned, we started the unit with a video chat with a fellow Freedom Writers Teacher, Cathy Cantu. Cathy was targeted by the community where she was teaching and using the Freedom Writers Diary. Her account of this attack can be read in the book Teaching Hope entry #89. During the video chat, Mrs. Cantu gave her account of the banning of the book and then my students were given time to ask questions. It was a firsthand account of an event where a book was banned and this brought the lesson topic to a level of reality in students' perspective.

Also, during this unit the Open Debate Activity on pages 134-137 of the Freedom Writers Teacher's Guide was used to dig into the debate of whether books should be banned as compared to the issue of freedom of speech as specified in the United States Constitution. An outline of this unit can be found at http://bannedbookunit.wikispaces.com.

I have been using the Freedom Writers Diary with my Saturday reading enrichment classes to offer students extra help with their reading and writing skills. We read selected journal entries together and students are given prompts to respond to that dovetail with the reading of the journal entry. Another Freedom Writers Teacher friend, Marcia Nelson, helped me with the reading prompts. Students then share what they write and we talk about the various topics. Discussions can be quite lively and emotional at times.

Most students have something to say about what they read in The Freedom Writers Diary. After the students write, they are asked to read their writing to the class. This often leads to further discussion and analysis of the dairy entry and the students' writing.

Erin Gruwell has been a guest speaker at our campus at the Worsley School in Fresno County's Juvenile Justice Campus located in Fresno, CA two times over the last ten years. Freedom Writers, Maria Reyes and Robyn Marotta, have also been guests at the juvenile hall. The Freedom Writers Tiffony Jacobs, Darrius Garrett and Lisa Shouse have addressed our students by video link.

These talks are televised to all the classrooms in the facility because only about forty students fit into our library where the guests actually speak. A group of students were brought into the library and video was projected onto a large screen. Students in the library could ask questions and students in classrooms throughout the facility email questions to the library to be answered by the speakers.

My students love to watch the Freedom Writers Movie. I show picture slideshows of all the Freedom Writers events that I have attended over the years. We spend a lot of time talking about the Freedom Writers and there are always many questions and opportunities to write.

My Saturday reading enrichment classes played the Line Game this year. This is the first time any of my students have played this game. Playing this game in classes where movement needs to be minimal because of the potential for violence has always been a concern. This concern turned out not to be relevant, the game was very effective and the writing the students produced was from the heart; it was amazing.

Another game I tried this year was Freedom Writers Bingo. I used Fruit Loops as the markers for the game. Vocabulary was studied and cereal was consumed. The classes had a lot of fun and expanded their vocabulary at the same time. It was a win-win.

The first Freedom Writers strategy I started using with my students was journaling. This approach has been instrumental in helping students to improve their reading and writing. Today each new student in my class receives a journal to use for assignments, to record their thoughts, to draw pictures, for their own purposes. Students take their journal with them when they are released.

A Freedom Writers Teacher colleague and friend, Scott Bailey, started a blog called *The Writing Exchange* and about six years ago he invited me to participate on his blog. We now develop writing prompts for each month of the school year. New writing is published each month and other juvenile halls and schools have also participated in the exchange. We all have our students write and each month each teacher submits their students' best writing to be published on the blog. The blog can be viewed online at http: //www.writeyourtruth.blogspot.com.

Below are some examples of my students' work:

Where I'm From

I am from a big family, where holiday meals are feasts.
From hard times any other day.
From seeing nothing but roaches in the kitchen.
I am from the "ghetto", where I learned patience.
From being laughed at every day for being the only white girl.
I am from a place where we fight,
But only for the respect that was never paid.
I am from a place where fights turn into murders,
And murders turn into wars.
I am from the track me and my brother built
In the fields of tall grass we would ride bikes to get away.
I am from clouds of smoke
That my family would constantly blow.
I am from my abused and neglected mother who is my hero.
I am from a well-respected man who is my father,
Later turned to a meth-head schizophrenic.
From broken bottles of a drunken step dad.
We are from new beginnings.
From joyous times at the river with my mom and step daddy
dearest.
I am from 6 hour floats with cases of beer.
With the homeboys I grew up learning to trust.
I am from 8 foot tall flames.
From bonfires where sparks touched the night sky.
I am from big dreams.
I am from broken hearts.
From young love,
Followed by broken promises.
I am from false hope my family gave.

I am from feeling guilty, for ending up just like them.
We are from the shame of being told,
"You will never be good enough!"
l am from my family,
Where We stand together and prove them wrong.

Where I'm From

I'm from rocks, chipped and splintered
From loving arms to a harsh, cold voice
From hot summer days forced to work
I'm from nights of no dinner because of mistakes
From bales of hay stacked like a tower

I'm from razor blades, silver then red
From days of hot tears streaming down my face
From insults screamed out of many mouths
I'm from dirt stained floors, and the smell of chickens
From arguments over religion

I'm from glass and shattered mirrors, shattered dreams
From the ammoniac smell of hair dye and insecurities
From dark eyeliner smudged across my eyes
I'm from bruised knuckles and the sight of blood
From depression and isolation

I'm from years of built up scar tissue
From bland meals of seemingly artificial meat
From the sharp sent of mace tingling in my throat

I'm from clenched fists of suppressed anger
From barbed wire

I can't change where I'm from...
But I can change where I'll go

Never Again

I think it is so hard to stay out of the criminal justice system because while kids are here, they don't learn anything while they are here. I mean yeah, they are away from friends and family but that doesn't teach them anything. They come back because they don't realize the wrongs of their ways, so they keep doing the same things over and over again. This is my last time here because I have realized how many people I have hurt living the lifestyle I was living. I hurt my friends and my family but most of all I hurt myself. I have learned many ways to cope with what goes on in my life and figured out why I did the things I did. I have people to help and support me so I can get out and have a new mindset and outlook on life and what I need to do to accomplish the goals I have set when I get out this time. I know what I want and need to do in life and that's why I will not come back to jail again.

Labels

In my generation everybody has a label. I am known as "The rich bitch" "white girl" "snow bunny" "Tweaker" or "white trash". People judge by what appears on the outside and by their assumptions. Most people who have labeled me those names never got to know me, the real me. They don't know what I've been through or the struggle I have faced. They don't know the demons I battle or the hell I've seen. Just because I am White doesn't mean I have a perfect All-American family. They don't know I lost my mom to breast cancer when I was ten. They don't know my dad is an alcoholic who drinks himself away and lives a bachelor life as if he has no kids. They don't know I've battled drug addiction for almost four years. They don't know I was once pregnant and had no option but to abort. They don't know I've lived almost seventeen years in fear and violence. They just don't know. But yet, they sit there and judge me by what they see. If only they got the time to know me. But that might not be good either...I push people away when they get close. I'm scared to be hurt again or left behind like I don't matter. I'm scared of a boy playing a good role only to get into my pants and go. I'm scared of reaching out for help because I don't want to be a burden. I'm scared of getting too close to someone only to be let down again. It's not easy for me to trust. I feel everybody is the same in one way or another. That's why I like being independent, fending for myself and only having to be responsible for me. I know it's not right. But I've been doing it almost my whole life.

Hi, and Goodbye...

When I reflect on 2015 I think of a whole year that flew by without recognizing where I was or where I should have been. I would like to say goodbye to that bewildered girl who was constantly dazed and confused. Damn, I was a mess. Every morning I welcome the beautiful day to the beautiful things I can provide. The thought of the day in Mr. F's classroom is "No matter how you feel — get up, dress up, show up, and never give up." This is the exact motto I would like to welcome into my life this year. Goodbye old tweaker friends. Hello estranged family. Goodbye grungy girl that I never knew. I never want to see you again. Welcome lost hopes and dreams! It's easy to picture myself going to college and getting degrees in psychology now that I'm clean. I welcome myself to the world this 2016!

My Name

My name is lost, wandering alone
A name broken like glass carved into bone
My name, a caged bird with clipped feathers
A name of an ill fate that'll never get better
My name was free at one point in time
A name that was bright like summer sunshine
But oh, now a name full of shame
An empty glass, spilled, there's no-one to blame...
Except for my name
My name is, and forever will be, a beaten animal
A name that is scared, afraid of all
My name has been set afire
A name shriveled, hung by a wire
Angry, angry, I destroyed my name
A name destroyed, and I the same
My name is a horrid beast
My true name is hatred unleashed

The lessons I use do not always have a Freedom Writers imprint or strategy, but Erin Gruwell, the Freedom Writers and the Freedom Writers Teachers have become a part of my thought process and are a large influence on who I am as a teacher.

Barb Fouts-Melnychuk

Leaving a Legacy Behind: So many months wasted!

February 23rd, 2016 and it was the third night of not being able to sleep. I couldn't get my mind to quit racing. It was 1:18 am and when the alarm clock playing Keith Urban rings at 6:30am the fatigue will feel like a collapsed building that I am trying to crawl out from under. I am crying quietly so as not to wake my husband. I hated it when anxiety held me hostage so once again I admitted defeat and got out of bed. Not only has this year been hard on me but the guilt I felt for not being there as a wife and parent, because of the impossible work load, has been crippling. The stress of the job has just slowly continued to rise, even though I am running on my work treadmill 60 hours a week. I watch the end line continue to creep farther and farther away from me feeling helpless and impotent.

I completed the familiar ritual of quietly getting out of bed, grabbing my journal and heading downstairs to vent. Venting about teaching grade 9 language arts along with 5 new subjects; Social 9, Art 8 and 9, and two courses I have created from scratch this year. The first new creation has been the new Flex block reading tutorial, that occurs Monday to Thursday, 20 minutes a day, with 10 -20 grade 7 through 9's together. Obstacles with this plan: find new and interesting resources, resources that aren't being used by anyone in the school already, resources for students 4 to 6 years behind the norm in reading and resources don't cost any money. I can do this - became my mantra as the teaching load seemed insurmountable.

Then the administration team wanted to reconfigure the way options were delivered at my school. So Anna, one of my brilliant co-workers, and I created #edmonton#6days. An option to break the misconceptions our north end students held about the arts districts of their city. National Geographic had voted Edmonton one of the top 12 summer destinations in the world and we were trying to help our students appreciate diversity within our community. The time it took to plan 4 field trips in 6 weeks for 60 students was staggering. An uninvited stressor surfaced as my teaching partner, Anna, was dealt with the cancer diagnosis of her father early in the school year, and it had understandably consumed so much of her world outside of school. This tragedy meant the logistical planning of all these field trips ending up in my "work-to-do" bin. As more speed bumps along the journey kept surfacing I reminded myself that it was only November and I knew success was just lurking around the corner.

The final addition to my teaching load was providing literacy supports to our integrated 109 English Language Learners and our 23 funded special needs during 4, 45 minute blocks a week. This literacy position was a new one in my school so again the learning curve was straight up with no template to follow. The changes to my teaching load, the creation of two new classes, the extra work while a colleague faced familial stressors were crippling at times, yet none of them were the demon on my back tonight keeping me from sleep!

Ironically the support of my husband made 60 hours a week very productive and I felt like all the new course creations and new subjects were under control. On the one hand it felt like I was handling this rigorous teaching load. The noose around my neck was tightening because all of these new responsibilities had eaten away my energy needed to implement the Freedom Writer philosophy of empowering students to make a difference.

Within our classroom we had successfully created a safe place using the Freedom Writers Diary daily, and the many games to engage and enlighten my students. But in the early hours of this February morning all I could focus on was how behind we were compared to last year! By this time in 2015 my Changents, as they had named themselves, had put in 146 service learning hours during lunches or after schools to improve our class and our school and had hosted a visit from an original Freedom Writer. Yet it was a year later and we had only completed 1 service learning project, bottle recycling for January and February. The assurance that we had completed at least one project was short lived.

The custodian revealed that my students recycling had been stolen by community members. We were the only group this had happened to in 6 years and Javier was so apologetic that I just felt sorrow and anger together. So now the monies we received from recycling for the end of the year celebration, were also gone. All these little pebbles in my shoes were starting to feel like rocks I could not fish out. Yet I persevered and I would sit at my computer 11pm each night thinking "okay now how do we implement the Freedom Writer philosophy this year?" I was stunned, overwhelmed and isolated while trying to make this vision a reality.

I remembered starting this year sure of successfully replicating the authentic service learning and writing experiences of the previous year. Yet it was February and I was 3 months behind. Another factor to our delay had been the 3 weeks of missed class time between October and December due to leadership professional development, facilitating professional development within my school, a student teacher who was diagnosed after our practicum with a clinical anxiety disorder and finally with my mom's diagnosis of breast cancer. Although the 3 weeks were spread over a two months I felt like the hamster on a wheel running every week to get caught up. All of these circumstances had created a blanket of fatigue that was getting heavier each week.

In December I thought I was over the worst of the hurdles as the first trimester for both the new option class and the Reading Tutorial option class had been created and implemented, my student teacher had finished and my mom made it through surgery with great news. "Cure" was the word the doctors were using for my mom's prognosis and I felt like I could breathe again, like the weight upon me was lifting. The easy breathing lasted about 3 days and then pneumonia hit. Out for another week straight and my resilience was gone. Over Christmas break I got enough rest and decided that we would find a way to give back even though we were 3 months behind my schedule. I went back to school with a new attitude and determination that we would find a way.

I told my students that we were ready to start our fundraising campaigns and asked how did they want to start. The resounding voices shouted "bake sales!" My Changents from last year's grade 9 classes had epic sales, raising $200 in an hour so this year's group was ready to meet the challenge. We formulated a plan and set the dates. But again we were not allowed to act but this time it wasn't because I was wearing to many hats. The administration told us to stop!

The new leadership option within our school caused a ripple effect for everyone doing service learning. Schools are living organisms and ours had evolved in a way that empowered so many kids while cutting off the limbs of my new batch of Freedom Writers. Instead of one leadership class in junior high there were now 7 leadership options.

This meant 7 other groups were doing fundraising for well deserving causes. There had been so much fundraising going on at my school that our student body was tapped out. There was so much fundraising going on that I wasn't sure we would even find a cause that my school had not already worked for. There was so much fundraising going on that I had been told by one of my administrators that I could not even start the next stage of giving back until the end of MARCH! A March start up would put my students and I six months behind the previous year's class. A March start up meant only 3 months in the school year to build authentic empowerment projects. I felt numb and did not know how to tell the students our efforts were on hold again, without seeing their eyes showing the doubt behind everything I said.

This night of not sleeping had become the norm and as I continued to grow more haggard, I gained more weight over December to February, and I felt my life slipping out of control. This February night, shortly after I had been told to stop all fundraising until the end of March seemed like it was the straw that broke my back. I was defeated and started to believe that the successes we had last year had not been because of my orchestration of students and community partners, or my ability to motivate my classes to reach great heights. The successes were simply that I had been lucky to have such motivated students and things had just worked! My sense of being empowered was almost distinguished and I was almost beaten down, not sure I would be able to get up this time.

The tears started to flow again as it was now 3am and as a working mom there is no "I am too tired" the next day. Not only would I have to be up for work in 3 and a half hours but after school I would have dinner to make, house chores to do, music and homework and then more nightly planning as I was always teetering on the ledge ready to fall at any minute with the variety of new subjects. My research article, based on last year's results, was also still not done and I was physically exhausted! I could not accomplish all that had but put upon me and I was breaking.

I started to pray and finally said "I SURRENDER!!! I CAN NOT DO THIS GOD I CAN'T" and exhaled. While sobbing I felt an answer surge from somewhere deep inside that said "It's about time!" The sobbing slowed and a shard of hope started to shimmer. The voice in my head said "ask the students what to do" and my ego was pushed to the sidelines!!! But to be so vulnerable in front of kids was terrifying. I did not feel I was as connected to this year's classes because of all the initiatives we had not completed. I was sure these teens would just hear a bunch of excuses not my sincerity and attempts to make things work. 9-2 and 9-3 would believe I was a fraud and that there was no hope. Yet the voice continued to whisper ever so softly that I had no other choice.

I went to school the next day frightened and as I entered the school I was reminded that there are days my students felt this scared. I remembered being grateful for this fear and my empathy grew with every step I took towards my classroom.

At the end of the lesson I stood in front of the kids and was brutally honest. I told them about the stolen bottles, and the fact that we were not allowed to start our service learning in the way we had planned until the end of March. I admitted I did not know what to do next and that tomorrow we would brain storm together what we should do. Every student seemed to sit up taller and pay more attention. The silence in the classroom was long-lasting yet not hostile and there seemed to be a calm that came over the class. As they were leaving Ailwin, a student I had taught in grade 7 and now again in grade 9 handed me a folded piece of paper.

I waited until the end of the day to open the note as our 1-minute transition between classes did not seem like enough time for more bad news. After school the note suggested a way we could give back starting immediately. It brought tears to my eyes and the shard of hope grew. I also received an email that night from Scott, a male student, who also had an idea of how to give back. The students had been the lifeline I had needed all along. The irony, my arrogance and my pride in my students hit all at once.

The reason my Changents and I had been so successful the previous year was that we had been true partners. Only 1 student did not do any service learning last year, and he had Asperger's Syndrome. Although he did not like the service learning compo-nent he took a leadership role within our class to the point he named our group the Changents. With such lofty expectations of service learning, the goal of improved academic results, the op-portunity to publish a research paper and the encompassing teaching load I had forgotten how much I needed my partners in this journey. With this new awareness steps to success started to unfold before me. The custodian found me in the halls shortly after my surrender to let me know that there was extra funding in the bottle recycling fund so the 2 months' worth of funds would that were stolen would still be available for my students.

I went home that night and tried to do my mom duties, but my husband picked up the majority of the work, because my exhaustion combined with renewed hope and hardly any sleep was taxing. My students still believed me when I said they were going to make a difference this year. I just had to believe it too!

The teens and I moved into action quickly – we booked our first bake sale for April 4th and 5th, before anything else was put on the school calendar and I decided if we were bumped again I was going to head to the admin team and put up a fight. I knew fighting to start our "Legacy Left Behind" project was worth all the expansive energy, even if it the loss of admin backing while I was applying for leadership position was a possible outcome. We planned, made lists and brainstormed ways to make the bake sale a huge success. I ended up missing school during the second day of our bake sale but the kids, and supportive co-workers ran it smoothly without me. We raised $380.00 and we are on our way. They had accomplished their first fundraising initiative and found their voice, their desire and the teamwork needed to leave a legacy behind.

We have since run into a few more glitches, such as Ramadan starting June 6th and ending July 6th or 7th. Ramadan is the Muslim spiritual celebration of the revealing of the Quran, which means fasting from sun up till sundown for a third of my students. So the start of Ramadan meant the celebratory dinner planned for the end of June would have to be bumped up before June 6th. We set the feast for June 5th, the Thursday evening so we could celebrate together. But the year's pattern of the rug being ripped out from under us continued. The grade 9 farewell celebration was set for June 5th bumping our Freedom Writer celebratory dinner. This time I did not lose sleep I went straight to my students. We decided we could find another event to celebrate together as there was no point doing our celebratory dinner before June 5th. We were barely starting our service learning and we wanted to accomplish something before we celebrated.

We made it through the district and provincial writing exams and the students excelled on the district assessments. I was surprised when I realized that we had been accomplishing more with their academic success than I had thought possible. With so many interruptions during the first 5 months I was sure they academic results would be lower than the previous years. We had used the Freedom Writer's Diary a minimum 4 times a week, and I had used daily journal writing to create authentic writing situations but I had lost hope in so much of my classrooms routines. I was measuring this year's growth to last year's students and not focusing on all our current Freedom Writers had accomplished in spite of the many setbacks. I was so wrong and the pride the grade 9's felt seeing how much their writing had improved left me speechless. The success in their writing had also empowered and energized my grade 9's. While most kids are shutting down with only 6 weeks left my students were just getting revved up.

The grade 9's are starting their book of life lessons for next year's grade 7's immediately. One of the grade 7 teachers has agreed to use it as a weekly reading and journal writing tool. My grade 9's are so excited to write their narratives and then to create questions for journal prompts like the ones we use with The Freedom Writers Diary. A true legacy. The grade 9's are also going to create presentations to educate our staff about "What Social Media Looks Like for Teens" after some cyber bullying incidents have occurred in our junior high, help create a school wide fundraising day to aid the schools damaged during the Fort McMurray fires, and building empathy presentations for our grade 4, 5, 6, 7 and 8 students to try and educate the preteens and teenagers about the impact and power of cyber bullying. Scott and Ailwin are spearheading the campaign to create Acts of Kindness around our school to improve our school climate.

The icing on the cake has got to be the questions I started firing out to the universe at the end of February and the answers I received. At teacher's convention I starting looking for any ideas related to social justice as opposed to just fundraising. Because of the questions I have made community partnerships to agencies that are empowering teens to make a difference through action not just money. The leadership teachers at my school have asked if we could collaborate this upcoming August so that the leadership students and my Freedom Writers will be working more in tandem empowering teens to act and start the ripple effect right in their own backyard. I have found The Secret Agents of Kindness, started by Ferial Pearson, and my teens are emulating her project and becoming part of the Secret Agents of Kindness movement. As soon as I kicked my ego to the curb and walked the talk of collaboration being a partnership between teacher and students, each taking the lead at different times, our "Legacy Left Behind" project has exploded.

Am I terrified we won't get it all done – OF COURSE!!!!! When the fear takes over I just remind myself to ask the kids for help and breathe. They always exceed my expectations and have for the 24 years I have been a teacher. The nights of sleeplessness have been replaced with nights of such excitement that sleep eludes me for a while but sleep now finds me much earlier than 3am!

"Alone we can do so little, together we can do so much" is the wisdom Helen Keller discovered along her path of collaboration with Anne Sullivan, her teacher and friend. Helen Keller's story was the impetus that made we want to be a teacher. 24 years into this crazy profession my collaborative journey of frustration, perseverance and ultimately service brings so much joy to my life that I look forward to the blueprint next year's students will draft with me.

Lisa Liss

LineGame Problems

When I arrived at my fifth grade classroom a couple weeks before the start of our school year to get it organized, I was horrified to see that everything I owned was stacked haphazardly in the middle of the room! This included 22 large plastic tubs of almost 700,000 bandages, plus years of materials! Whew…I had work to do. About 6 of my former students showed up to work in the garden and even offered to stay to help me arrange my room! Looking at it with fresh eyes, I decided to make my room even better than it had been in the past. Together we moved all the bandage cases, the tables, the boxes and more. Excited about the change in my room, we began to set up the tables. Arranging the students' folders, I made sure to include the permission slips for the Freedom Writer Diaries.

Twenty-eight years of teaching and counting, and I can truly say that each year is a blessing and a challenge! This year followed the most challenging group of students in my teaching career. It was a breath of fresh air to listen to my 2015/16 class as we discussed what self-discipline is. I casually mentioned to them that self-discipline is when they remain in their seats and listen to me when all they want to do is to go outside and ignore me. I smiled as I looked around the room at the 32 serious faces looking like I said the weirdest thing ever. "You know, if I gave you the choice, how many of you would get up and walk out instead of listening to me?" Incredulously, I saw no hands raised! That moment, I knew this class was different.

The FW permission slips had come in and we began to read the Diary entries. After only a few short weeks, I felt this class was ready for the line game. My questions started with easy ones, "Stand on the line if you like pizza… Stand on the line if you have a pet…" The students seemed ready for the more difficult ones.

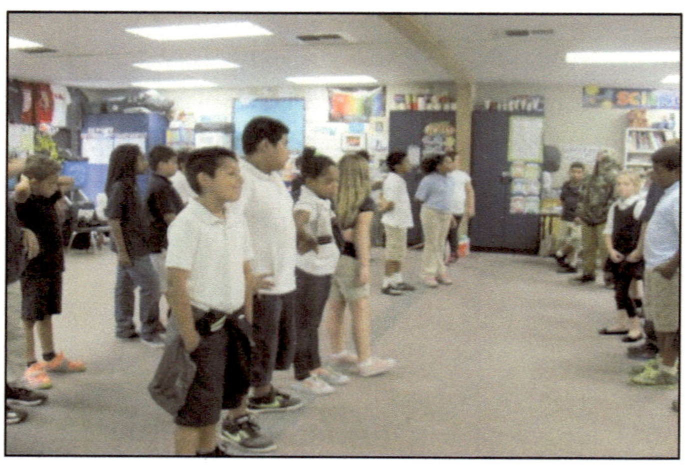

My first hint that something was different, was when 20 of the students remained on the line when I said, "Stand on the line if you live with both your biological parents." Actually, there are about 12 who live with both parents, but they were shy at first. (Usually there are about 6-10 who are on the line for both parents living with them.) The questions moved on to the harder ones, "Stand on the line if you feel drugs are a problem in your life." (22) "Stand on the line if you have ever been in juvenile hall." (1 and 1 more who did not go to the line.) "Stand on the line if you are afraid to sleep at night." (24) "Stand on the line if you have ever gone to bed hungry." (24) "Stand on the line if you know a relative who has been in jail." (27) In previous years, I've had students stand on the line for seeing someone killed, losing a parent by violence, and more.

At the end, one young boy was crying (the one on the line who had been to juvenile hall), most of the class rushed over to hug him and comfort him. I knew that the line game as well as other classroom activities, were working, we were becoming a family. A few days passed and things continued looking up until my principal contacted me. "Mrs. Liss, one of your parents called, Ben's Grandmother, and is upset about something called The Line Game.' I explained to Dr. Simmons what the Line Game is and we talked for a few minutes. I immediately called "Ben's" grandmother. We had a great conversation, or so I thought. She explained to me that Ben and his brother were living with her after their father and mother had both had drug issues and had neglected them. She went on to say that the day after the line game, Ben came home and refused to do his homework and was very angry with her. The more we talked, the more I tried to re-assure her that Ben's opening up to her is a good thing; that together, we can help him talk about his feelings and become more aware of ways to work through them. I offered to talk to her any time before or after school and gave her both my personal and school email addresses.

I thought everything was going well at that point, but it was only the calm before the storm! About a week later, Dr. Simmons called me on the way home one evening and told me that a group of parents had gathered at the projects and was angry about The Line Game. They wanted to know what I would be doing with the pictures I took. What would I do with the information I gathered? Why are the diaries not allowed to be read by the parents?

What right do I have telling them that what their children wrote is private and "secret?" Luckily, after spending 4 years with an evil principal and 3 years with a crazy principal, I now have a principal who supports me and knows that it takes courageous conversations to have students open up productively. Dr. Simmons alerted me that the parents had been meeting at the projects and wanted him to force me to stop any and all FW activities. He told me he let them know that would not be an option. He did request that I give students a story starter for their diaries and not read the book until we could have a meeting with the parents. Dr. Simmons then told me that the parents wanted to read their child's diaries. I told him that I would not agree to that. Although he was surprised, he already knew what a difference my faith in my students has made and told me he would be there as support, but that I could tell the parents this. He asked me if it were my own children would I feel the same way. I told him that as they were elementary students, yes. Regardless of their age, I think they need to have privacy. I told him that I wouldn't read my own child's diary unless I felt that they were getting into something dangerous and I needed to keep them safe. Dr. Simmons told me that he had already discussed this in detail with our district's Assistant Superintendent, who asked if he felt that my intentions were honorable and righteous. He said he knew that I only had the students' interests at heart and that he can honestly say I was doing what is right. The feeling of support gave me the courage to readily agree to the meeting for the following evening.

The day of the meeting, I discussed with my students that some of their parents wanted to read their diaries. I reassured them that I still did not want to share their diaries and still felt they had the right to write what they felt. I told them if they didn't want their parents to read their diary to write a note asking their parents to respect their privacy. I warned them that parents would then have to make the choice to honor their wishes or not. More than half my students wrote notes and I stapled them to the cover of their diaries. The remaining students agreed that they didn't care if their parents read it. One boy summed it up well, "Dad and Stacy, please do not read my diary. It contains my own personal thoughts and really, I don't know why you would want to read things that I want to keep to myself. I am entitled to write things without you reading them. I hope you will honor my request and not read my diary. Thanks!" Luckily, his parents agreed and didn't read what he wrote. Three parents did read their children's diaries. I told them that one of the reasons that I do not allow anyone to read their thoughts, is that they need a safe place to write what they are experiencing without fear of repercussions. I explained that as long as what they were writing didn't let me know of anything that was currently harming them, that I wouldn't do anything with what I read.

It felt like a small lynch mob as the parents entered the room. Most of the ones who complained the mightiest did not come to the meeting. I know that fear is what guided the parents to gather together, and fear caused them to lash out. Fear of whether I would call CPS, fear of whether I would call the police, fear of losing their child. The one grandmother in particular who instigated the initial uproar, really just wanted a sounding board. She is overwhelmed with raising two boys after thinking she was finished raising kids. She wanted an audience and to be heard; I was just a convenient scapegoat. Dr. Simmons had reached out to the projects community and gave them someone who would listen. This was a first for them, but it also opened up their feelings of power. Had they come to me instead of to each other in a community forum, these questions could have been addressed earlier with less animosity. Things quickly got out of hand as one after the other shared their impressions of what was going on in the classroom.

Gathering quotes from FW conferences and arming myself with copies of FW lesson plans, I began to prepare to have the meeting. I decided to have the Line Clip from the FW movie ready as well as to start them with a clip from the "Pass it On Commercials." At each seat, I had some Fruit Loops and a vocabulary page. I ran off copies of all my materials and waited for the meeting to begin. One parent walked in, the concerned grandmother of Ben. She glared at me and took a seat. Then Arthur's mother walked in with a baby in a stroller. About 10 minutes later, Arthur's dad came in as well. A few minutes after this Ms. Neighbor, the mother of two of my former students, arrived. It seems that Ms. Neighbor, having already listened to their concerns, would be the spokesperson for the parents. I began with the Pass it On clip and then showed the parents how to play Fruit Loop Bingo. None were willing to play a round, but it did break the ice. I sat at the table with the parents and listened as they expressed their concerns. I explained that the Line Game and Journals were ways to bond and that it gave their children a safe place to express their feelings. It also gave me a chance to "talk" personally to each one of them every day. I assured them that nothing their child told me would be used against them. I explained that if their child were in any danger that the first step I would take would be to talk to Dr. Simmons. We then discussed the diaries and how I firmly believe that parents should not read their child's diary. I explained that even Otto Frank had not read Anne's diary until years after her death. Dr. Simmons stepped in and said that he saw how the diaries helped my students last year and that several students have asked him if he could make their 6th grade teachers do the same thing.

Ms. Neighbor asked how parents were supposed to know ahead of time that we would be reading the FW Diaries and doing these activities. I informed her that all parents were given permission slips at the start of the year. None of the parents remembered this until I showed them their signatures. At first, Ben's grandmother said that she wanted to remove her permission. I told her that this was her right. Dr. Simmons had already told the parents that I was not going to stop the curriculum and that their only recourse would be to remove their child from our school. To alleviate their concerns and fears, I apologized for not letting the parents know before I played the Line Game and told them that in the future I would hold an FW conference the first week of school to acquaint parents with the program and alert them that their children might be opening up regarding their feelings. Arthur's father seemed to really understand at this point that the program would only help give the children a means to open up. He left confident that this is an appropriate setting and style to be used. Dr. Simmons told the parents that what they were getting from me was something that it could take years of therapy to achieve, and that they were fortunate we were starting young. He said the curriculum is first rate and they were lucky to be benefiting from it. Ms. Neighbor perused the curriculum guide and asked a few questions. Things went uphill quickly and the parents started to understand the reasoning behind the games and activities. Dr. Simmons told Ben's grandmother that she had to make her decision right then on whether to continue or remove her grandson. She quickly agreed to keep him in my class. I also agreed to let the parents know if I became aware of anything that might affect their behavior at home, and for them to do the same thing for me. I ended the meeting with a reminder that I am at school early every morning and leave late every afternoon. I gave them each my business card and wrote my personal email on each as well. They assured me that they would all be writing me that evening. As of yet, none of them have written or contacted me since. We are back doing our FW "thing," and life is back on track. It takes Courage to Stand up and it takes courage to help a child. I'm willing to stand and have courage!

Richard Mellot

For my students

I've been a very bad boy. I pushed the limits, I challenged my students, I challenged my administrators. I'm ok with that. Everybody needs a little nudging. I'm an instigator, an agent for change. You will not forget me. I will not forget you. Here's a taste of my life.

I got involved with the Freedom Writers Foundation (FWF) quite by accident, when I contacted them about doing an interactive videoconference with my special education class. I was teaching at Roosevelt Middle School in Glendale, California. However, because of my deep interests in the use of educational technology, I had been working on interactive videoconferencing with teachers in Manizales, Columbia, Singapore, Bakersfield, California, and Austin, Texas. My goal was to enrich the environment of my classroom, by making experts, authors, and successful people appear on the screen.

I had just picked the FWF off of the Net randomly, because I was looking for authors to interview for my class. I sent off an investigative email, and got a positive response. They wanted to know more about the format, and since this was in the same area as I was, the Los Angeles basin, only about 40 miles away, it seemed like a simple request to me. When I talked to the person in their office, they seemed interested, so we started talking about the logistics. They'd never done a long-distance interview with anyone, so to them it seemed too technically difficult, but I assured them I could get them help. I talked to a colleague I knew from an educational conference, where I had been presenting on a different topic, and he volunteered to help. This was the way Glen Cornish and I partnered up to do the very first Freedom Writer's Foundation interactive videoconference.

After I discussed the project with my principal, she said the idea was "too good to keep to myself," and she encouraged me to talk to the English Department. I talked to the chair of the department, who agreed. Together we met with the English Department, explained what I was doing, and we asked teachers if they would like to participate. Everyone thought it was cool, especially when I suggested that we could invite the whole school.

To make a long story short, I wrote curriculum and lesson plans for all the teachers. Then, we got permission from almost all parents to show the PG-13 movie. With the permission granted by the FWF, and an investigation of the uses of films in the classroom, we showed the film "Freedom Writers," to the whole school, classroom by classroom. This was the way we used the Freedom Writer's movie as a jumping off point for lots of discussions, writing, and book reports. Students and teachers prepared questions for the upcoming videoconference, and submitted them to me, the host of the event. I chose some of them to be presented to the actual "Freedom Writers" from the audience. I set up a microphone for the audience, so we could ask our questions live. The students were all getting excited.

I was the host on the school end, and we put our set up together in the School auditorium. Glen was down in the Freedom Writer's Foundation building in Long Beach. When the day came, we set up the conference between our two little laptops, using Skype. We also invited a third party, Ms. Joy Lewis and her class from a high school in Binghamton, New York, to join in. At that time, three party conferences were about the top capacity of

Skype, so we had to plan it very thoroughly, as it complicated for those days. We also had a technical difficulty to overcome in the school auditorium, which didn't have a network access. We were forced to use a hundred-foot network cable, plugged in to a classroom wall, out the window, and across the pavement to the front door of the auditorium, where we covered it with rugs.

This was a fairly complicated arrangement in itself, but it came off with only a couple of hitches. Once we had the conference parties all present, there came a howl of feedback, and we had to scramble, since it was happening in front of an audience of over 500 students. I went to the door, so I could hear Glen on my cellphone, and we decided we would break the connection, and see if we could isolate the source. We discovered that it was coming from the Texas school. Later we learned that someone in the New York high school had left a microphone open, and it created a feedback loop. We had to cut the connection, and it did get me yelled at by the vice principal. I still remember her howling at me to get back in and control the crowd, and I had to tell her to be quiet, I was on the phone trying to sort it out.

However, we were able to keep in touch with the Freedom Writers, and they were troopers while we figured it out, making it a little easier for the audience, who could see we were still with them. The students got a little loud, but settled down when the conference restarted. We were able to ask the two Freedom Writers questions, and it was a great time, as they talked about the now familiar story of how it all happened to them. Many of the students got to ask questions and the answers were often of an inspirational nature. So much was learned, it is hard to quantify, but I know it's burned in my memory as a great achievement. I think positive memories are really the basis for greater motivation, so I felt like I had made an impact in many lives.

Since then, the FWF has been doing videoconferences as an increasing part of their outreach, and I'm happy to say I had a hand in helping them develop the model.

We did this for two years running from my school, with more success since we had experience on the possible pitfalls. In the meantime, I did other related videoconferences, with two different holocaust survivors, and a catholic priest who was a friend of Miep Gies, the Dutch woman who hid Anne Frank and her family in the famous Anne Frank home, now a historical museum in Amsterdam. I also did interactive videoconferences with two authors who wrote a book together from Africa and the US, using SKYPE.

My little special education classroom was a very innovative place, where I used educational technology to help students with disabilities overcome their learning differences. Since I was being creative, and often pioneering new approaches, there was no previous data on which to rely. This was somewhat problematic for my teaching evaluation, and it got me in a lot of trouble with a stodgy administrator. She was always asking for data-driven, direct instruction, and eventually, she gave me a bad evaluation based on my lack of use of "standardized formats for education."

I thought that was very ironic, considering I was at the cutting edge of use of technology in a classroom. Many of my students were writing illustrated book reports in PowerPoint, as well as doing mathematics lessons online, and studying history by doing webquests, a form of Internet research. Many of my parents were crowing that their autistic students were so happy. I shrugged it off as the price to pay for leading, and took my disciplinary year of evaluation with a grain of salt.

Then, I got the call from the FWF that I had a shot at filling a vacancy at their summer Institute that year, so I got to go get trained by Erin Gruwell, and to become a part of their team as a Freedom Writer Teacher. I told my administrator, who gave me permission to attend, and covered my summer school classes with substitute teachers, and I attended the Long Beach session. It was such a rush to meet other innovative teachers, many of whom I'm still in contact with, via social media. We were introduced to the Freedom Writers, did workshops on techniques, given lesson plan books, written by Erin Gruwell, and I got to have a dance with Erin herself at their dinner party for us. We got to go to the Museum of Tolerance, where we were entertained and educated by the director himself, who told his own story of redemption. We were also given inspirational speeches by several holocaust survivors, stories of their survival and the suffering they witnessed.

Finally, we went to the Paramount Pictures Studios, and were given a private screening of the Freedom Writers movie. All of this had such a deep and lasting impression on the teachers, as it was a recreation of the motivational events that had inspired the Freedom Writers themselves. Many of us were moved to tears, even though we'd seen the movie many times at this point. It created a bond that is unbroken to this day.

One of my last years of teaching in California, I also got invited to participate in the previews and reviews of their series of books, "On The Record," a Scholastic Books collaboration with Erin Gruwell as an advisor, on middle school books for motivating struggling readers. I was on a team that reviewed text and content, advising the editors on presentation to a classroom of struggling readers. As a result of this consultation, I was presented with a classroom set of the non-fiction series, which told the stories of many individuals overcoming difficult situations, told in a very personal and yet academically valid format, which I used for my own classroom with interesting results. When I retired, and moved to the Philippines, I donated it to a small public school that used it for English Language Instruction.

Again, I was given a bad evaluation for not using standardized educational approaches, which at this point, I decided to just let stand, I was tired of fighting the system, so I took an early retirement as an option to escape disciplinary action again. I had begun a teaching side job at an online university, and for four years, I had been working two jobs, which also contributed to my burnout. My mother's passing away was the last straw. However, I felt vindicated that I had lasted as long as I did, defending my students from an uncaring educational system. I felt like a smaller version of Erin Gruwell, and I was able to see a way forward.

I left California, I left the USA, without shame, and have continued working in education, to this day. I've since volunteered on a national level with the Autism Society of the Philippines, and taught English at a private school in Thailand. My latest news is that I've just been awarded a job as an English Lecturer at a private college, where I'm going to be contributing to the use of innovative instructional approaches, using educational technology. I was actually hired because I'm a proven innovator. So, life for me, as a Freedom Writer Teacher goes on, and I bring that spirit of reaching for the light wherever I go. But I'm still a bad boy.

Anne Schober

Close Your Door – Open Your Heart

When I became a Freedom Writer teacher in July of 2007, my life as a teacher changed beyond what I can accurately place into words. Erin Gruwell taught me to respect each person I meet and take the time to learn the stories that surround my students. She taught me to believe in myself as a person, educator and cheerleader for the at-risk youth that God graciously placed in my care, and the college bound students that needed guidance. She taught me to teach with my heart.

When I returned to school in August, I was given a class of students that had placed lowest on the entrance exams; a group of 25 students from all different backgrounds, ethnicities, and economic backgrounds. Some would be the first in their family to graduate from high school, while others came from affluent and prominent households. What I had in front of me was a "mix" of kids who quickly took up my entire heart. And, what I had in front of me were kids who learned differently from any other group of students I had encountered. And, I had no idea how to teach them.

I began by incorporating Study Skills hoping that this would help them succeed as they began their journey in high school. Together we learned different study techniques, how to use the library and the computer system to perform research for their various classes, and implemented the help of outside tutors and teachers to help with math and science. Our hour together was spent learning what I thought they needed to succeed. However, something was missing.

My "Mix" kids needed more than just study tips. They needed me to hear their stories, to understand them and to accept them for who they are, in the here and now. I learned this the hard way. One morning, my kids walked into my classroom with heads down and grim expressions.

"What is wrong?", I asked.

"Today is Friday, that means we have to do math and library stuff. I hate this day!"

And, one by one, they all agreed. They hated coming to my classroom! I gathered them all together and they began to voice their concerns.

"We are getting so bored."

"I go from one class to the next and it is all the same thing… listen to the teacher, do a worksheet, take a test. The same day in and day out."

"I thought this class would be different."

"I heard you are a Freedom Writer teacher, what does that mean?"

I listened. My heart ached. I had forgotten so quickly what Erin had taught me: To teach with my heart. I went home and quickly decided that I needed to change in order to help them to succeed. And I began with the Toast for Change.

One of the most life changing events I experienced while at the Freedom Writer Institute was the Toast for Change. It allowed us to put our past behind and put the future ahead while proclaiming what we wish to change. It was powerful because we publicly exclaimed our thoughts and it allowed us to also share our failures and successes. I knew this is where I needed to begin.

I ventured into my classroom over the weekend to prep for our Toast for Change which would happen on Monday morning.

I moved all the desks to the outer walls and decorated the room with streamers and posters. In the front of the room stood a lone table filled with champagne glasses waiting to be filled with sparkling cider. My heart was racing… I knew that this celebration would just be the beginning.

Monday came, and I began. "I want you to take one of these glasses of sparkling cider, and I want you to make a toast. We are going to make a toast for change. What that means is from this moment on, every voice that told you "you can't" is silenced." Slowly each student took a glass, took a turn, and spoke their toast for change.

"I am going to graduate from high school and go on to college. I will be the first in my family to do that."

"I am going to start doing my homework and stop making excuses."

"In the past, I have been rejected by others because of who I am. Thank you to all the "mix" for not giving up on me and believing in who I am."

One by one, they continued their toasts and that day proved to be just the beginning of our newly formed family.

In our second year together, I noticed their angst more and more. They were bored and not as successful academically as I had hoped. They struggled in many of their classes and their self-esteem was waning. Everything we had worked on for the past year was slowly fading away. Something needed to change.

My aunt and uncle, who had previously lived in New Orleans, were visiting and during our time together, they spoke passionately about the atrocities and the aftermath of Hurricane Katrina which had happened a few years prior. Listening to them,

I knew my students would benefit from hearing about the devastation and the ongoing problems in a place that holds so much history. They agreed to come in and the "Mix" were transfixed on their every word. It was after they left that things became interesting.

"We have to do something to help the people in New Orleans!"

"We need to go help build homes, or bring food. We need to go help!"

Their excitement was contagious and I quickly bought into their energy. I went to administration and asked if it were possible for us to go to New Orleans to help rebuild after Katrina. And, while they thought it was a great idea, the "higher ups" would not allow us to go, naming "Post 9/11" as the dominant reason. I went back to the class, passed on the news, and saying they were disappointed would be an understatement.

"Well, nobody needs to know that we are going! We can go after school is over!"

"Yea, we can leave the day after school is out and nobody will know! Come on, Ms. Schober, let's do it!"

I knew this was not a good idea, but the rebel in me knew it was the best thing for these kids. They needed this. They needed to feel needed. They needed to feel important. They needed to change the world.

And so, I closed my doors to my classroom and we planned our trip. We held meetings outside of the school day so that I could say, when needed, that this was not planned during school hours. We held secret parent meetings. We planned car washes at Burger King and Walmart, held bake sales and created a letter campaign where the kids asked for money to go toward their trip instead of Christmas or birthday gifts. They were energized and I could see them change before my eyes. They each signed a paper stating they had to pass each class in order to go on the trip and they each needed to raise $500. The turnaround was unbelievable. Their grades increased, their attendance was flawless, and the trip was now a reality.

The school year came to an end and the next day, fifteen of my students, along with my daughter, two parent volunteers and I, boarded a plane from Baltimore to New Orleans. Nobody at school had any idea… it was our little/big secret. We landed in New Orleans and the kids were mesmerized by their new surroundings. As we drove to the church where we were staying, they could see the devastation that surrounded them. They saw homes that were evacuated and boarded up with numbers painted on the plywood stating the number of lives lost in the home. They saw boats toppled on dry land and cars abandoned. This was five years after Katrina had landed and parts of New Orleans looked like it happened yesterday. We met with Habitat for Humanity about our work schedule and the next day we would begin to help rebuild New Orleans. The "mix" was ready to get to work.

The weather was hot, humid and oppressive. But, the kids never complained. Over the next five days, they helped to build five new homes for those misplaced. They met the people who would live in the homes, listened to their stories, and worked with their hearts through the hottest of days. They hammered more nails than I care to count, hung drywall, installed roofing, and hung Tyvek. They formed blisters and some came close to heat exhaustion, but never complained. We left our mark on New Orleans and five days later we flew home, changed.

I went into school a few days after we landed and asked to meet with administration. I knew that I could possibly lose my job, but I also knew that the transformation that I witnessed in my students was too dramatic to not share. We met, they listened. I was reprimanded but praised. I was "written up" but cheered because I had left with fifteen students and came home with fifteen adults who were ready to change the world. I accepted the reality that what I did went against administration and the rules that I was to follow, but I knew instantly that it was all worth it. And, so did they.

My "Mix" kids stayed with me for all four years of their high school education and they did "big" things. They raised $16,000 and built a playground for a school in Nashville, Tennessee where the average family income was $5,000. They helped mentor freshmen students who were just like them, and they wrote a book that told their stories of heartbreak, loss, hope and success. Because of them, a new class was added to the curriculum based on what the work they did in New Orleans. And, because of them, I no longer had to close my door.

Marcus Strother

Getting in trouble for me

We had just gotten back from our 16-hour drive from New York. During the drive we shared stories, expanded on the knowledge we had just gotten from the conference we attended and worked hard to hit every note in the hip-hop and R&B songs we played. Driving into work Monday morning, I was ready to share our experience with my colleagues and other students. What I wasn't prepared for was the moment that would change my life forever.

My Monday morning at work started in its typical way. Good mornings were shared with students and colleagues. I handled hall duty in the usual fashion and I dealt with a few unpleasant situations. After a few hours of this, I noticed one young man walking my way. I knew he was coming to me because he was in my mentor group and we had built a pretty close relationship. He did not attend the New York trip, so I figured he was coming to get the low down on how the trip went. This was not his intent. He stepped to me with a confusing look on his face and that is when it came out. "Why didn't you tell us you weren't coming back?"

At this point, it was my face with the confusing look and he tried his question in a different way. "Why didn't you tell us you got fired?"

I immediately attempted to act as if this was a young man that didn't know what he was talking about. I brushed him off with a simple response and sent him on his way. Even though he walked away without a fight, I should have known that it wasn't the last time I would hear from him about this. I taught them how to use their voice. I taught them to stand up for what they believed in. In my own mind I suspected that I needed to practice what I had been teaching. I knew I needed to find out what he was talking about, but it was March, I had time, so I thought. By lunchtime, the news had spread and colleagues were inquiring. It felt like I was being questioned at every corner of the school building. Students were whispering and I was lost. I really had no clue what was going on. By the time I made it to the lunchroom, my stomach was in a knot. One student came to me and showed me a petition for me to stay in my position at the school and it had over 500 signatures. Now I was really beginning to think that I needed to find out what was going on, but my boss beat me to it. My radio went off and it was my boss calling me in to her office.

As I walked in, she stated, "Marcus, what is going on?" Now, to be honest, I had a few responses that I didn't share. This was my opportunity to find out myself, so I remained professional and I looked at her with the same earlier confused faced and shared that the students believe I'm being fired and they're pretty upset about it. It was at this moment that I knew my students were right. The woman's face completely changed and she handed me my evaluation. First of all, this is not how my overview of my evaluation should have gone. Secondly, this was not a scheduled meeting. It continued to get more interesting. While I read through my "EXCELLENT," (yes, I had received the highest measurement possible on our evaluation scale) evaluation, I heard these words. "I have decided to let you go and move in another direction. Could you sign your evaluation please?" Now, take a moment and think about being in my position. I had just come back from an amazing trip with my students, questioned by my students and colleagues about being fired, and was now given an excellent evaluation, with confirmation that I was being asked to step down from my position. As I took a moment and looked at my boss, my mind shifted to my father who had been in a union for a long time. Although we were not in a union, I knew that he could give me some guidance on how I should handle this. I had no prior conversations with my boss that stated there was concern about my job performance or that I would be let go. "I am not going to sign this right now. I need to speak with my father first." I made this statement and walked out of her office thinking that I needed to figure this out. What I didn't know was that the students and parents were already a step ahead of me.

As I walked to my office and called my wife to let her know what had gone on, she became immediately supportive. We talked about all that had gone on and decided we would talk more when I got home. I went through the rest of my school day dodging questions and attempting to shut down any worry that my students had about me leaving. What you will find out was that my attempts were a complete failure.

I got home from work and as I always do, I kissed and hugged my wife and kids. I sat down for a moment and my phone rang. As I picked up the phone, one of my co-workers was on the other end and began telling me that I needed to be prepared for tomorrow because the kids were not happy about me being fired and they are not going to go to class. I asked him what he meant by "not go to class" and he said, "They are going to refuse to go to class until they know you get to keep your job. Marcus, these kids love you!" My immediate thought was that it wouldn't be that big of a deal, until my phone rang again and again, until the call was my boss asking me if I heard about what was supposed to happen tomorrow. As we talked through this, we felt that we would be able to contain the issue if it came up. Again, the power of youth organizing was happening and I was not prepared.

Tuesday morning came and it was time for me to go into work. I listened to my music, thought about how the day would go and prepared for another day of changing lives. I walked into the school building that day and I immediately knew that something was different. I walked down the hallway and my students began walking up to me saying, "We doing this for you Strother." "We love you Strother." "Don't worry Strother, we got your back." I wanted this to be smooth, whatever "this" was going to be. I dropped my things off at my office and headed out to do hall duty as usual. The students started coming up to me more and more. I found myself checking my watch more often than usual. The anticipation of what this might look like started to get to me. There it is, that first bell that told the students they needed to go to class and had one minute to do so. And then it began. The second bell rang, which meant that all students should be in class.

Here were my emotions at this time: I stood in the hallway and my heart was pounding so loud that it was all I could hear for a moment. My eyes began to water because of the tears that were coming, no matter how hard I would hold them back. My breathing became heavier than usual. I looked down the three hallways I could see and I paused for a moment before I realized what was really happening. In my mind I thought, this is not happening right now, but it was. Sitting down in the middle of the hallway floors were hundreds of students all confessing to the fact that they were not going to class until they knew that Strother would keep his job! For the next 55 minutes, administrators, teachers, hall monitors and school resource officers attempted to get these students to class, but they would not go. The word was spreading that there was a riot happening at our school. Parents began to show up. To their surprise, there was not a riot happening. Once the parents found out why their student was not going to class, most of them began to support their student. What we soon learned was that there was one particular mother who had a student at the school and she had allowed the students to organize this sit in at her house, with her help. With all of the calls that were going out, our district office Superintendent showed up at the school. By this time, the bell for the next period had rung and we thought that the sit in would end at this point. The bell for the next period rung and again, the students were refusing to go to class. At this point, even more students got involved because others began to hear about what was going on.

By this time, we knew we had to gain some control and our principal convinced the students that she would hear them out if they all went into the auditorium. I found out how organized they were at this point because the students had already appointed 6 students, 4 young men and 2 young ladies as their spokespeople. They agreed to move into the auditorium and the students began walking that way. A strange thing happened during this movement. A strand of firecrackers went off in a trashcan. We never found out if that was from a student or an adult, it felt like an attempt to create hysteria. The students did not let that change their direction. They were focused and moved right into the auditorium. Once we had them in, the principal walked over to me and stated very abruptly, "You need to help us get this under control. Talk to them" I looked back at her and said, "I'll say something, but I think they have their mind made up." I raised my hand to get the students attention. They got very quiet and all I could fix my mouth to say was, "I appreciate what you are trying to do, but you have to go to class." Immediately there was a hush in that auditorium and one young lady stole my heart and made me realize that my students were ready to get in trouble for me today. This young lady stood up and yelled out at the top of her lungs, "But we love you Strother!" I broke down. I looked at the principal and she knew that I was done. She stepped in and attempted to calm the students. She again pulled the spokespeople in to her office, but they stood their ground. My cell phone began ringing uncontrollably with calls from my wife, mother and father. As I stated earlier, it was being called a riot, but there was no riot. More parents were showing up and now the local newspaper was at the school and they had put out a quick website blurb about what was happening. The Superintendent and other administrators decided on a plan. They announced to the students that they had busses coming and that the students had two choices. They could either return to class or go home on the busses that were being offered. If they refused to do either, they would be suspended for disruptive behavior. At the time they thought of this idea, I am sure they thought it was the best plan. What they didn't expect was for all of these students to leave school and with it being so early in the day; the Superintendent and other administrators had given the students time to think about what they would do next. That is exactly what they did. The students left school and came up with their next plan.

Once the students were out of the building, I went to my office to take a moment, but it wasn't given. Local news outlets were reaching out to get information from me. Colleagues were wanting to talk about what had happened, saying things like,

"This stuff only happens in the movies. This is crazy." My family was all reaching out to make sure I was okay. I did as much as I could that day to keep things normal, but it was about to stay in a state of not normal for a while. Later that afternoon, the administrative team was called into the principal's office. It was at this time that we were informed that they had been notified that the students were going to be doing a march tomorrow morning down the main street of our town starting at 6:00 AM and ending at 7:30 AM at the school, where they would continue to demonstrate what they wanted. As an administrative team, a plan was put together, but I quickly knew in this meeting that I was being shut out. I listened and prepared for the next day. In my mind, I wasn't sure I was prepared because I was the central focus of what was going on and everyone wanted to know my thoughts. I finished the day and immediately went home to my wife so that I could talk with her and get some type of comfort. The stress was beginning to get heavy.

On the next day, I did my usual with a different mindset. I listened to songs on my way to work that soothed my heart. I prayed differently. I smiled and I cried. This was very emotional for me. As I got to the school and walked in, the emotions were high with everyone. I walked into the cafeteria to find every administrator in the district; elementary, middle and high school were called to work at our school that morning to help with any issues. I became the immediate outcast. Only one of my administrative colleagues spoke to me, almost as if they were all told not to and he just didn't listen. The call came over the radio that the students were almost here. They had really done the march. I later found out that the students convinced a local church pastor to use his church insurance to give the students a million dollars worth of insurance to do the march, which were the city guidelines. The students began walking to the front doors and they were immediately ushered into the auditorium. There were parents with them. The parents seen me and came up to me and told me how much the students loved me and that they were going to fight for me. One of the young ladies, who was one of the spokespeople for the students had to be sent to the nurse's clinic because her feet were so swollen from walking and the cold. I was so overwhelmed and humbled by all of what was going on. The students had planned to go to the emergency board meeting that had been called and they asked me to come speak at a community meeting that would happen before the school board meeting. I did go and speak at this community meeting and shared what I knew, which was nothing. The principal and the Superintendent both showed up at the community meeting, but did not address the community. I went home after the community meeting because I did not want to cause more problems by showing up at the board meeting. However, I felt like I was there because my phone and text messages were going off telling me how all of my students were speaking out during the public comment portion about me. The meeting would last almost 3 hours because of the number of students and parents that spoke on my behalf.

I made it to work on that third day, but I would not make it long. The stress from all that was going on began to be too much. While sitting in my office, I had an appendicitis attack. My wife took me to the hospital and I had to have immediate surgery. I was out of work for three weeks, but I do know this much, my students did not stop fighting for me. They came to the hospital and checked on me. They called my home and checked on me and by the time they were done, they had caused such a movement that they attended 6 school board meetings speaking on my behalf, created enough noise that our local newspaper wrote 11 articles in three weeks, created an internet buzz throughout our area that other schools were talking about it, and SAVED MY JOB! My students, or as I call them, my babies SAVED MY JOB and SAVED MY FAMILY. I knew the moment I got the phone call at home that the school board voted against the principal's recommendation to let me go, that I would always be about my students first. I knew that I had found my purpose. Mark Twain said that the two most important days in your life are the day you are born and the day you find out why. I found out why and my babies showed me that as long as I loved them genuinely and did all I could for them, that they would be willing to GET IN TROUBLE for ME!!!

Henry Wright
A better life through education

Can you get into trouble or be rejected for following the law or by doing what is right? I did. Encouraged by Civil Rights activists who risked their lives for equality, I followed the words of John Lewis. I got into trouble. Here's my story: A law was passed by our federal legislatures. As I followed the law and took my stance, I was intimidated to cease my actions. In the fall of my junior year in high school, there was a big push for integration in the public school systems in the United States of America. The states met some resistance, especially in the southern states where I resided.

Even though the desegregation law passed, a majority of Caucasians in the southern states made it known felt that African Americans were infringing on their rights. Not only did white people find it unpleasant that a few black students were attending their school, surprisingly some of my friends also found integration unpleasant and did not understand the need to have change in our country. My school district was trying to be proactive with integration of schools by allowing a select few black students to apply and attend the previously Caucasian only schools.

One hot sunny August morning, I walked down the dusty dirt road with my friends. We were chatting as we walked. As we approached a paved road that was perpendicular to the dirt road, I began walking toward the paved road. My friends asked, "Where are you going?" I told them that I was going to school. Someone stated that I was crazy. Another person stated that I was going the wrong way. Someone else student stated that I was really going to the store.

As I walked this paved road each step became harder and harder. My feet felt heavier and heavier because I knew at the end of this road was the bus stop to go to the new, formerly all white kids', school. What was different about this bus stop is that I would be the only African American at this bus stop. No other African American had stood at this bus stop to go to school. My deodorant was working overtime. As I came closer to the bus stop, I could see cars passing by and I saw boys smoking cigarettes. There was a smell of peppermint candy. These boys were dressed in oxford shirts, dress slacks and penny loafers. This was a little different from what I wore because my outfits had been purchased at a department store and not a specialty store.

I was asked where I was going. I replied, "To school." Someone asked, "Aren't you at the wrong bus stop?" I inquired if this bus went to this particular school. They replied, "Yes." Someone asked what grade was I in. I stated, "Eleventh." The bus arrived and I climbed inside. I walked about half way down the aisle and sat down all by myself. There was no National Guard, mother or father. I felt very vulnerable. The bus began to move to the next stop. The bus was filled with quiet chatter and glances toward me.

At the next stop, an attractive Caucasian girl got on the bus. She greeted her friends and then she noticed me. She stated that there was "a damn nigger" on the bus. As we arrived at the school, a tall man with a pointed nose directed us to the gymnasium. I endured two years of rejection by most students and faculty at that school. There was a hand full of African American students at this school. There were no African American teachers at this school. The only African American adults I saw were the cafeteria and custodian staff.

The cafeteria and custodian staff were proud of us for making history by being the first African Americans at this school. They were the friendly faces during each of these difficult days at this school. Of course, a few years later the school district had full integration of all their schools.

I didn't want to be a teacher! After high school, I joined the United States Air Force where I worked as a Disbursement Accounting Specialist. I took some college courses that would fit in a bachelor degree in Business Administration. I had no interest in becoming a teacher. Once my service in the United States Air Force had come to an end, I enrolled as a student at the University of South Carolina and studies in the School of Business Administration.

Once I received my Bachelor of Science in Management Science from the University of South Carolina, I worked for a variety of establishments. I have been a manager for a retail outlet, worked as a computer programmer, worked as a delivery person/salesman and supervisor of a sales group. I was between jobs when my wife suggested that because I loved children that I might enjoy being a teacher. Me? *A teacher.*

So, I made an appointment with the school district. I talked with the Assistant Superintendent of Schools for my county about becoming a teacher, He asked if I had a college degree. I told him that I had a bachelor degree in Business Administration from the University of South Carolina. He inquired what I was thinking I wanted to teach. I told him that I thought that I wanted to teach courses in Business Administration. This nice gentleman came from behind his desk and he sat next to me. He stated that he didn't want to discourage me but if I really wanted to be a teacher that I should come on board as a middle school teacher. I took the few required courses and began my career in teaching.

My first teaching assignment was in an urban elementary school where I taught 4th and 5th grade students. It is during this time period that I worked to receive a master degree and an educational specialist degree. The school's population was about 65% free and reduced lunch. I taught at this elementary school for ten years before I became the Parent Involvement Coordinator where I was able to do frequent home visits. The school counselor and I implemented a program to distribute coats to the students for the winter. I started a program to improve on-time attendance and late attendance to school for our school. At this elementary school, I was chosen as the Teacher of the Year one year.

After years of being at the elementary school, I left to become an administrative intern at a middle/high school for students with behavior problems. During the summer after my year at this school, I was selected to serve as the English/Language Arts teacher for a new program to help with dropout prevention for high school students. This program witnessed an average of 50 students per year receiving their high school diplomas. While at this school, I was selected to participate to the Freedom Writers Institute in December, 2007. There are approximately 450 Freedom Writer Teachers living in every state within the United States, seven provinces of Canada as well as several other countries around our world.

Our county had some budget cuts and a program, which had great success, was discontinued. I transferred back to the alternative school for students with behavioral problems. I implement activities from the Freedom Writers Diary Teachers Guide, daily. Also, I use activities that students will have to use Higher

Order Thinking Skills (HOTS). One of these activities involves students finding facts about a person and making inferences about the background of the person that they research.

As a professional teacher, it gives great joy to share and discuss with my students information that is new to them. I see my students as an extension of me in that what is my ceiling/zenith in education is their floor/foundation. With the information that they gather, they can continue to learn and become lifelong learners.

I am the youngest of six children in my family. I have always been the adventurous one in the family and my community so I did not follow the road of others but I have tried to blaze new trails.

Does this make me a dreamer? Yes, I am a dreamer. If you can see it when no one else sees it, then you will probably believe it when no one else will believe it. For the last two years of high school, I went to a different high school than my brothers and sisters. I went to a college that was different than the ones that my siblings attended as well.

My undergraduate degree is in business administration which was new to our family but today, I work in the field of education where I help students of all races to drink the cup of knowledge to its depth. Frequently, I have been considered as the Jackie Robinson of my family.

I have used the Freedom Writers Methodology in my school. We have used the line game to allow students to see how much they have in common. Guest speakers frequent my class. What do a sheriff, mother, domestic violence survivor, owner of a semi pro football team, state senator, United States Army recruiter and Latino business owner in common? They have been guest motivational speakers for my students. My students have gone on many field trips. One of the most memorable field trips was to Atlanta to serves as PAGES for State Senator William Ligon. Another field trip was to Savannah, Georgia to see Erin Gruwell where we spent 2 hours discussing the concept of writing.

We have had the privilege to attend the Scribblers Writers Retreat on St. Simons Island, Georgia. My students listened and mingled with writers from around the United States who talked about the importance of writing. My students published a journal in 2008 titled "Saying It PLC Style! The Golden Isles Teen Journals." In 2009, my students published their second journal entitled "Saying It PLC Style! The Golden Isles Teen Journals Volume 2." Both of these books were edited by a professional editor, CoCo Harris. Soon, our Volume 2 will be republished.

Do I continue to get into trouble? Yes, I get into trouble daily because I present to my students a view of a better life by educating them rather than letting them come to school and do nothing. The students that I am entrusted with are students who have gotten into trouble at their schools or they have gotten into trouble in our community. Many of our students have been incarcerated in juvenile detention centers and some have been abused physically, emotionally and mentally.

Frequently, I share about the two roads and how choosing my path has set me apart from some of my high school classmates. During my junior year in high school, my English teacher required us to read the poem, "Two Roads," by Robert Frost. This poem lets students know that you don't have to keep doing the same thing and expect different results. This poem allows them to realize that it is alright to try other things and it allows us to be acceptance of others. Oftentimes powerful words give us the freedom to 'get into trouble.'

*Torbjørn Ydegaard, with Kathrin Schaller, Dennis Röben and Frederik
Wärn Pedersen*

Freedom Writers in the Arctic

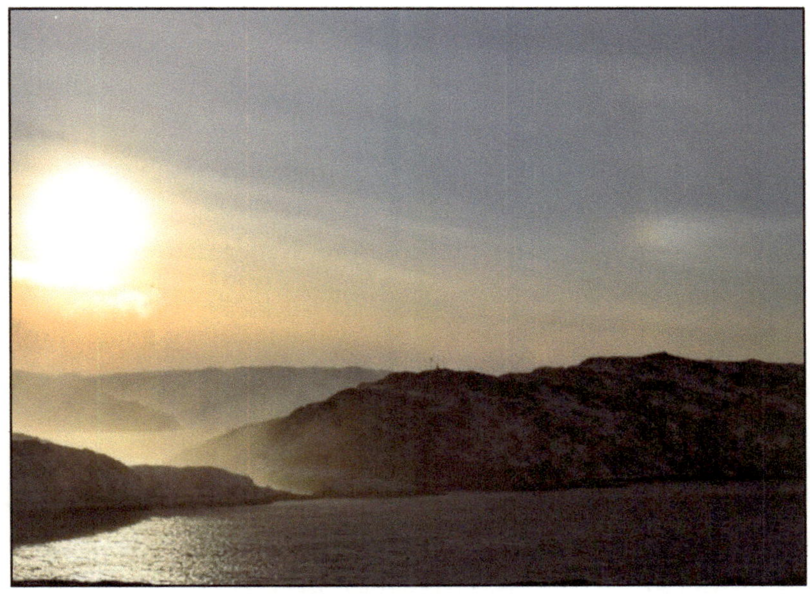

Hi Torbjørn, one of my students, doing her internship in a small
village in Arctic Greenland, emailed me, *I have a question for you…
We have started our Freedom Writer-project with the adult-group (although
the language-problem makes it a bit difficult). Every day some of our participants hand in their diaries for us to read. Today we got a rather upsetting
story. A young woman wrote how she was raped 11 years ago – and that she
afterwards gave birth to a boy. We know this boy from our teaching in the
school. I didn't know how to react. The lady came to me after a lesson and
asked if I had read her entry. 'Yes' I answered. 'How did you fancy it?' she
asked. I didn't know what to say, and I am not sure what I said. Torbjørn,*

I felt sorry that for the woman and her son, and for my students that had to face such a story. However, I was not surprised. Even though things have gone much better the last decade Greenland – as part of the United Danish Kingdom – is after all housing tremendous social problems: problems with poor housing, alcohol, drugs and sexual abuse. Therefore, when my students were working with the Freedom Writer methods among young people who have dropped out of their educations and moved back home to their villages, without having a job, those problems had to turn up.

I am not blaming anyone for the misery. Not the Danish colonial power that ruled Greenland from the beginning of the 18th century, nor the Greenlanders or their government. I have travelled intensively in Greenland over many years and I know the history of the land. Whoever ruled the country always did so with the very best intensions – ranging from protecting the population from the materialistic outside world to giving them all the opportunities of that same world. And if these good intensions were guided by the very best of knowledge of the time being, how can you blame anyone for things going wrong?

Well, things often went wrong in Greenland. But a lot of things also went well. In the middle of the 19th century the Greenlanders were the most alphabetized people in the world, they were reading newspapers with colored pictures (the first in the world to bring colored pictures) – two numbers per year and brought up along the coast in qajaqs! Gradually they were introduced to democracy, while traditional hunting and fishing from qajaq and dog-sledge have remained the basic of the economy in the small villages – only Greenpeace's campaigns against the use of seal-furs and the recent years' climate-changes form a real threat to traditional life.

I answered my student as this:

Hi. First of all, it is great that you ask what to do! When that is said, you neither can nor shall be a psychologist. You can ask, if the lady wants to talk about her story – and if so you can meet her with empathy. Probably you cannot report the rape to the police after all these years.

And as my wife said, when I showed her your mail: "This is exactly what the Freedom Writers is about – to make people tell their story and through that empower their life".

Keep on – you are doing a great job!

Totally I had six students out-placed in Greenland, in three different villages. They both taught primary and secondary levels in the local school as well as groups of adults with very little connection to neither education nor job-market. The adult groups were organized through what is named the *Nuiki-project*, that aims at motivating and qualifying drop-outs for skilled training. From what my students tell after two months in Greenland, Freedom Writer-methods seem to be adequate and highly usable also in the Arctic:

Dennis Röben

LineGame in Greenland

We are located north of the arctic circle, early in the year 2016. The school is small, but still a big building when it comes to how few students that have classes here. The school is un top of a hill, not far from the harbor in the small village with 120 citizens. One would think that in a small community like this, there should be a great unity with good relationships and a prosperous society, but that is unfortunately not the case.

This could be because the citizens are divided in small groups, which depends on their origin, education, work, family and much more. This creates a gab and a lot of arguments amongst them.

One could wish that the students would leave their indifferences and arguments outside the school's front door, but that is unfortunately not the case. As a teacher it can be difficult to get the students to focus and help them develop in class, when there is so much else taking their motivation and energy. The different issues of the small society, becomes a problem for the students´ possibilities.

These obstacles are especially seen during the classes for the adults from the village, these classes are every day except weekends, for 3 hours, and here you would meet people who are as different as they come.

Right before our departure to Greenland, my comrades and I were introduced to the Freedom Writers philosophy by one of our lectors, Torbjørn Ydegaard. After we saw the small groups and conflicts within the group of our students, we decided that it would definitely not hurt to try that angle with them, even though the situation was complicated by communication problems, such as a lag of a proper translator or translation aid.

It took a little time to find the right tool to start with and at last my partner and I chose the LineGame.

We started with a careful approach and easy questions, like the following:

— *Do you have children?*
— *Do you have a job?*
— *Are you born here?*
— *Do you have a husband or wife?*

Nobody had ever asked them to present themselves, show others who they are or acknowledged them for precisely the person they are.

We were surprised how fast and happily they opened up and the LineGame became a frequent visitor in the lessons, the following 7 weeks of our stay, 10 times at all.

We often combined the LineGame with Mindmaps, which the students had to fill out before or after the LineGame.

Despite of the fact that all of them had known each other for their whole life and lived in the same little village, where everybody knows everybody, we could observe how the group grew together and that the members began to support each other.

After the second week, we allowed the students to ask questions and we would participate with them. We were well aware of the risks of that, like too personal or harsh questions or a loss of authority, but the students were gentle and respectful. Their questions were mostly related to their everyday life, feelings and emotions regarding recent events in their society.

The main problems in the village were the addiction to alcohol and other legal and illegal drugs and a lag of education in general. After about three weeks, we calculated that the risk of being rejected and losing the fragile connection to our students, were small enough to move on to the more serious questions, regarding the main problems in their society. They had accepted us and we were no longer total strangers.

The next three weeks went by and the two main themes of our LineGames were their own social role in society and their plans for their very own future. Here are some of the questions:

– *Do you have a role model?*

– *Do you think everybody needs a role model?*

– *Are you a role model?*

– *Do you want to be a role model?*

– *Can a group represent a certain list of qualities and cultural norms?*

– *Do you think that a group like that could be a role model?*

These questions were followed up by different exercises and a Mindmap about what a role model is and who can be a role model.

Other questions were:

– *Do you know what you want to do after you finished this adult education?*

– *Do you need to move to fulfill that wish/dream?*

– *Are you scared by the thought of moving away from your hometown?*

– *Are you afraid of the risks and the responsibilities you are going to face?*

The questions about their wishes and dreams were combined with an exercise that we called "motivation cards".

The main purpose of this exercise is to get the students to define the reason why they are in school and to motivate their education. They should define why they are going to school, what they want to reach with their education, regarding their family and establishing their own lives. Every time they feel unmotivated, or feel like not going to school, they are supposed to look at or think about this motivation card, so they can find support in their own wishes for their future.

The journey has shown us, that even if you could use just one element from the Freedom Writers philosophy, there is huge potential for a great result and a good experience. There is a great possibility for a good social development as well as learning relevant progress, using these tools.

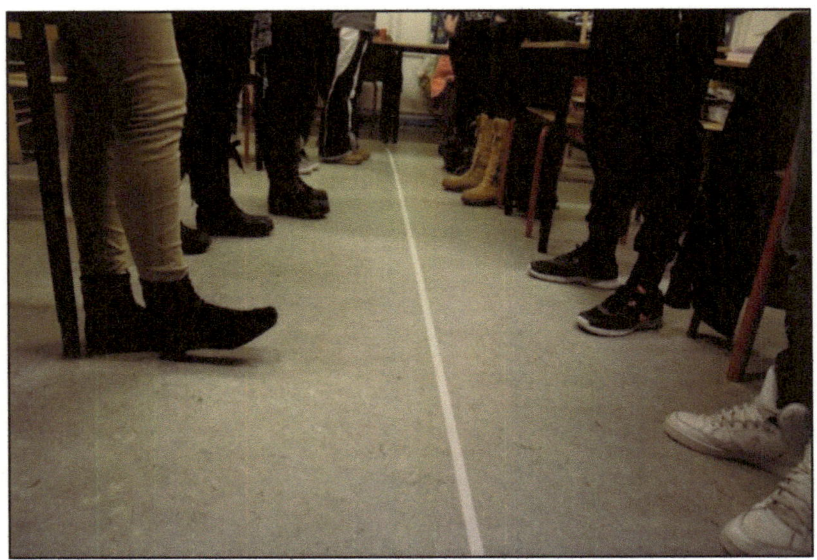

Frederik Wärn Pedersen

Use of Freedom Writer methods in Kangerlussuaq

In my internship as teacher-student I chose to go to Greenland. I have an inner power towards helping others, as well as seeking personal development. Greenland seemed the perfect destination for exactly this.

Before departure I took part in a Freedom Writer-course. This could that be one of the methods to get closer to the kids I would meet and to create a safe environment for their development. One-and-a-half month in Greenland is not much time for change, but luckily are the Freedom Writer methods exactly so concrete and tangible that they can be implemented also in a short course like this.

I used the LineGame as an icebreaker in grade 6/7 where the children are around the age of 12. I was convinced that with the right questions this approach very soon would loosen them up and create a bond of trust between us. Therefor I made up 20 questions that I thought fitting for the age-group having in mind their cultural background as Greenlandic children. It worked out perfectly. But it was a transcendent experience for some, and they chose not to participate. These children are maybe those which would have the most benefit to feel themselves as part of the community. Once "again" they were excluded. Between the pupils and me.

Same approach was used with the adult group. Here everybody took part in the Linegame and again with the feeling of bonds being created.

The adult participants are partners in a project called NUIKI, which is a one-year course taking place in many villages all over the country. NUIKI aims at preparing the participants for further education. The target group is very broad when it comes to age-span, but common for all is the lack of simple academic skills and especially lack of personal competencies for taking part in an institutionalized education – and in the society as such.

With the NUIKI-group I used the OpenHead-exercise, where they would write their inner goals and thoughts inside the head and their outer circumstances outside of it.

I started by showing my own example, as I felt would give them trust in the task and to show them that telling your own story in our common forum is okay. As these people often carry around heavy thoughts that they typically don't share with others, many of them had a hard time getting started. Maybe they are embarrassed by their own stories, and often they have a very low self-esteem. I gave them some examples and they began to feel themselves more comfortable with the exercise. At the end several of the students presented their OpenHead and their reflections on it. I have a clear feeling that they found this both comfortable and at the same time transforming. Especially pleasant for them was the fact that someone in their surroundings wanted to listen to their personal story and help reflect on it.

All this made one of the participants wanting to write her own story in a more extended version. She was academically well-situated and didn't need very much support before moving on. She wrote a really beautiful story about a Greenlandic young woman at the age of 22. And she told how excited and challenged she had been being forced to reflect on her life as she had to tell it in her own words and by putting these words pen to paper.

Kathrin Schaller

Freedom Writers in Greenland

For my internship during the teaching education in Denmark I got the chance to travel to Greenland and teach a group of 15 young people between 17 and 29 years old for five weeks. Even though time was short, I was convinced that they would benefit from the Freedom Writers methodology. Just like Erin Gruwell's group, our students were the ones, who had failed (or had been failed by) the school system and no one believed they would be able to finish an education and contribute to society. They were used to follow and obey and to be stuck in a box that just didn't seem to fit right. My goal for the internship was to open up this box and the world for them, to make them think for themselves, believe in their own abilities and make smart decisions for the future. And what approach could be more fitting than Freedom Writers?

However, arriving in the small Greenlandic settlement it quickly showed that there were a lot of differences between the situation in Room 203 and the one I was standing in. My students didn't have the problem of being divided or too diverse, they were very homogeneous and dependent on each other. Understandably that is how it has to be in a small society like the one they grew up in, but it didn't fit to the expectations of a modern education or workplace. An introduction where I asked "What makes you unique?" lead to 15 same answers: "I want to learn Danish and English." Furthermore, our students weren't outspoken, challenging troublemakers, they were very shy and quiet, not comfortable talking in front of other people. And another difference: I wouldn't be able to teach them in their mother tongue Greenlandic. So while they were supposed to deal with personal development and other topics, that some of them never had thought about before, this had to happen in a foreign language, which some of them didn't speak on a basic conversational level. So it became apparent quickly that I would have to adjust some of the strategies and activities used in Freedom Writers.

My own requirement was to use at least one Freedom Writer activity (FW) in every lesson. Freedom Writer activity meaning tasks that where embracing 'Ms. G' 12 Secret Sauce Ingredients' while aiming at personal development and giving a feeling of empowerment to the students. Following I will describe some of the activities I used and the experiences I made with them.

One of the major tasks as a teacher is to create a safe and inclusive classroom environment for all students, because it is a prerequisite for learning. I could observe a positive effect of FW on how comfortable the students felt in class and in expressing their opinions. Activities like 'Coat of Arms', 'The Peanut Game' and 'Walk-and-talk' (from Cooperative Learning) were encouraging for the students to express their own ideas without being judged. Simply giving them tasks where there was no right or wrong answer was almost revolutionary for them. It was a big challenge for them to comprehend that we were not aiming for a specific solution. They didn't seem quite comfortable with it in the beginning, but as time went by and I kept encouraging them, the enjoyed it more and more.

After one week we had a movie night, where we watch the FW movie. The fact that the story was real and we were able to show them the actual diary written by the Freedom Writers made a huge impression on them. I could sense an energy in the room that hadn't been there before. They could identify themselves with the characters' challenges and we had a good talk about what the Holocaust was with them. But my personal, unexpected highlight of the evening was when one of the students asked if they could write diaries. Of course they could! They each got their personal diary and on the next day I could collect the first stories. Though writing the diaries was difficult due to the language, many made a point of writing about their daily life regularly. Some stories were very personal telling about bad experiences from the past and I must say I was surprised by how much some of them were able to open up in their diaries. But I could clearly sense that they liked to tell their story and be heard, because some came after classes and asked "Did you read the diary? What did you think?" It brought us closer together. Unfortunately, some students never handed in anything and

A dinner party where they made traditional Greenlandic food for us was the perfect occasion for our 'Toast for Change'.

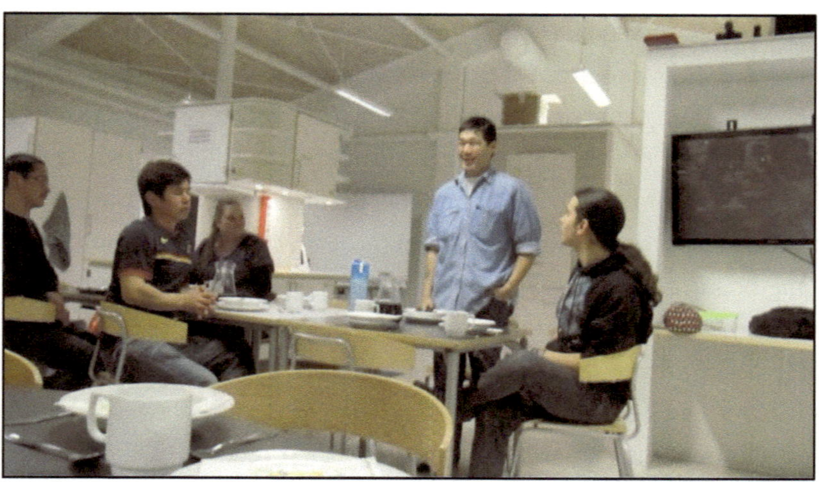

Many focused on learning Danish and English again, but some named personal and professional goals, which was a good step in the right direction. But actually the biggest learning happened for them by standing up and saying something in Danish in front of everybody else – and getting applause for it. That's why I decided to assign short oral presentations for every lesson for every student to have a turn during the rest of my internship. One of my shyest students gave the following speech: *"If you really want to move on then do something about it. Show them what you can do, even if you have not been so good, just believe in yourself. If you keep moving, it will be much better and better."*

Also the Line Game had a big effect. I used many questions suggested by Torbjørn Ydegaard in *Alle har en historie IV* and supplemented with some relevant questions for Greenland, such as Step to the line if '… you like hunting' or '… you or somebody that you know has or had a problem with alcoholism?' They said that it was very good that the questions were formulated in the way "you or someone that you know". The atmosphere started very fun and cheerful, but throughout time it became more serious and I could see that they were really thinking about the questions and their answers. Most importantly they were able to take their own decisions comfortably, because they didn't have to speak. So they were not just following the class leaders like they normally did. Afterwards we sat in a circle and every student got a matchstick. We saw how easily it could be broken. Then everybody added their matchstick to a pile and we tied them together. No matter how hard even the strongest guys in the class tried to break the pile, it was impossible. This was a good way to illustrate what the Line Game already had shown them: We have more in common than we think and together we are strong.

When we talked about the Line Game afterwards many said that it made them remember or miss friends and family, so it was natural to continue with a 'Wall of people we want to thank' instead of a 'Wall of dreams'. Our students wrote cards like this one:

Dear parents (Dad). Thanks for all. You have made me to what I am. From my birth onward you have met many dangers and good things, without surrender and without leaving us. You have given me many advises and taught me many things. Hope you are satisfied with me. Without you I might not be here. <u>To smile</u>. You are always by my side. You mean a lot to me.

As I mentioned earlier I had to open their eyes to their own strengths and originality, so I used an activity called 'Draw a tree' that is not specific to FW. The students had 2 minutes to draw a tree individual, no further explanations. This was the result:

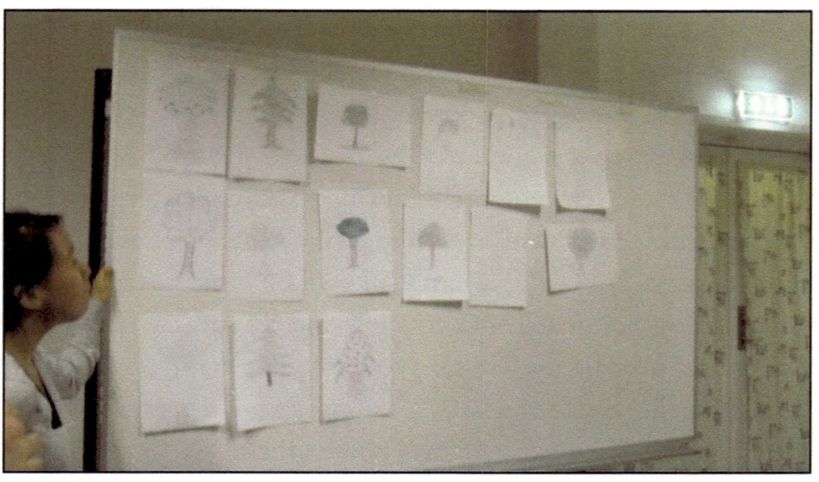

15 completely different trees, every single one beautiful and special in their own way. *"We are not all the same, we are unique"* is what the students remembered afterwards from this activity. Afterwards they each had to write a story about their tree, which was quite fun, because many of them had only seen a real tree once in their lifetime during a study trip to Denmark.

Summing up I could observe how FW slowly made the students open up, dare to speak their mind and rediscovery the strength they all had inside them. This became obvious in the feedback I got form them as well: *"You gave me courage." "Writing about myself made me feel like a new person, I feel relieved." "You gave me many ways to defend myself." "I have learnt that I am not alone with my goals."* I believe that some of the skills they have learnt from this FW course will help them in their future education as well as private lives.

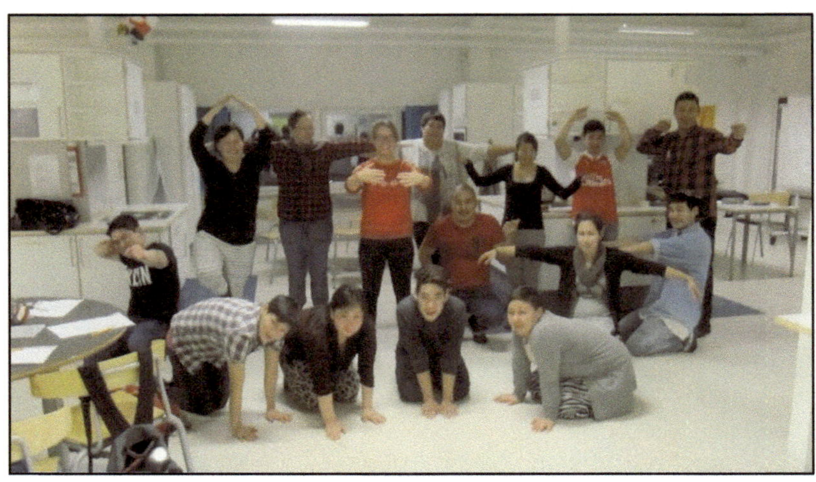

We used a lot of roleplay and drama as well.